THE CHARON CLUB

GINA M. BRIGHT

To Georgeane,
thank you for
your interest
in the nurses'
story.

Gina M. Bright

RIZE

CONTENTS

The Charon Club
text copyright © Reserved by Gina M. Bright
Edited by Abigail Efird

Published in North America, Australia, and Europe by RIZE.

Visit Running Wild Press at www.runningwildpress.com/rize Educators,
librarians, book clubs (as well as the eternally curious), go to
www.runningwildpress.com/rize.
ISBN (pbk) 978-1-955062-71-8
ISBN (ebook) 978-1-955062-72-5

To those of us who dared to care.

PART 1

VIRAL REDUX

HALLOWEEN, 2020
Porky's Farm, Clinton, North Carolina

The clouds swirling over the gravel road receded as the five pickup trucks skidded onto the grass in front of the nursery barn. Tucker Abbott saw them from his upstairs bathroom window where he had been sitting since feeding the litter of piglets before dawn.

Maybe it was dehydration, he thought, from all the visits to the toilet over the past few days that accounted for what he saw when the men stepped down from their vehicles. He knew they were men with their egg-shaped bellies and thick arms brought on by middle age. But their faces were covered, and not just with handkerchiefs protecting their noses and mouths from the dust of the long road leading up to the farm. He blinked again.

Tucker hated that he had to open up his farm to the public now, on Saturdays, like this one, for the past three years. Porky's Farm, as his father named it for his favorite cartoon character when he inherited it in the early 1940s, boasted the

1

best furrow to finishing product in all of North Carolina. Tucker continued the tradition when he took over in the early 1980s.

But when soy bean farmers could no longer offer their grain wholesale to the pig farmers, after they lost the lucrative Chinese market when the tariffs came, Porky's farm could no longer nurture the piglets into the 300 lb. specimens that always demanded medals at livestock competitions and top dollar on the market.

A decent profit was to be found, Tucker discovered, in selling the piglets right after they were weaned around 15 lbs., and only fed with soy bean for a day or two instead of the months required to grow to full size. Tucker needed to sell 40 piglets a week and these Saturday buyers helped him reach that number.

He was down at the barn now.

"I'm Tucker. Tucker Abbott," he extended his hand to the largest of the five men.

The man said something as he shook the farmer's hand.

"Come again," Tucker replied.

"My apologies," the man said as he removed his hood and gestured to the other men to do the same.

He could see the farmer was uncomfortable. "It's Halloween, after all, Mr. Abbott. We's just haven some fun."

"What can I do for you fellas?" Tucker asked the man who never did give him his name.

"We woan to buy some of your fine pigs. They real little, right?"

"Do you have a cage for them? They need to be secure for transporting."

"We got our own and plenty of straps for 'em."

"I have just about a litter's worth. Just been weaned from

their mothers yesterday. Even had their first taste of soy beans before the sun rise today."

"We woan two of 'em each, if you have that many."

"Sure do, fella. That'll be $60 per piglet."

Tucker Abbott was pleased. That meant $600, almost half of what he used to get for full grown ones back in the good days. But he felt like he needed to be honest with the men before the transaction was completed.

"My piglets aren't as lively as they should be, on account of the heat, I believe. Our Carolina days have been well over 80 degrees. Unusual indeed."

"We been even hotter in Alabama. We thank you for your frankness, farmer. We know you have the best piglets around."

The farmer thought it was odd that these men had no questions about how much soy bean the pigs needed as he took their cash. And then what he saw after they loaded the piglets in their trucks was even stranger.

Four Georgia and one Alabama plate all ending in the letters: JD. Then all of them placed their white hoods back on.

"They must be Klansmen who like a shot of whiskey now and again," Tucker Abbott said as he hurried back to the bathroom.

ALL SOUL'S DAY, 2020
Florence, Italy

Sophia had been wide awake since 4 A.M. She knew what today was. Giorno dei morti, the Day of the Dead. Italy's official holiday to honor those not walking the earth any longer. If she had paid tribute to all who had passed through her life, Sophia could have filled a banquet hall.

Instead, she set one plate at the table, the tradition in Italy, for Ricky who should have been here with her.

Late 1992
New York City

Sophia was meeting Patty, her good friend from her Bronx childhood, for a nice meal and just one glass of wine. But the gnocchi in creamy carbonara was so good and Patty was so happy she had met the guy of her dreams, again, the glass turned into a bottle. Normally, that wouldn't be a problem, except Sophia needed to be on duty in a few hours.

By Christmas, Patty and Angelo were engaged and the official party was scheduled for New Year's Eve. Sophia was invited, of course. Patty asked her to be a bridesmaid. Sophia could not remember bringing in the last few New Years. And she was beginning to feel like she wanted to, even though there was not that much to be hopeful about.

New Year's Eve, 1992
New York City

She knew that popping in at Patty's soiree for "just one drink" would lead to five or six. So she stayed in and watched *When Harry Met Sally* on TV with two slices of pizza from Tony's, around the corner on 3rd Avenue.

She called her old friend, an ER nurse, who she knew would be home, after the movie was over.

"Kathy. Hi. It's Soph. I think I'm ready."

"Your timing is impeccable, Sophia. But tonight's as good as any other. It's usually standing room only though."

"It's time, Kathy."

"The closest one to you is the Methodist church on 86th and Park."

Kathy had been in recovery for years. She was the one who smelled the wine on Sophia's breath that night after she had dinner with Patty. Sophia received an admission around midnight from the ER, and Kathy transported the patient up to her unit. The patient was masked and so was Kathy until the patient was isolated in a room to rule out tuberculosis.

As Kathy lifted the man onto the bed from the stretcher, Sophia, maskless until she removed his, met her in the middle pulling him over.

Kathy said, "Light as a feather. Your patients are always so easy on my back. Sophia, you should think about taking it easy on your liver, hon."

Kathy often called people that. She could not shake off the Baltimore in her even though she had lived in New York City for years.

Sophia was nervous as she walked up to the church. "Who would've thought I'd end up here, New Year's Eve, 1992?" she said to herself.

It wasn't that Sophia drank all of the time. This night, for instance, she had cappuccino with her pizza and movie. It's that when she did, one or two was never enough. And lately the drinks were getting closer and closer to her shifts.

She read the sign inside:

"A new life for a new year.

Meeting downstairs, 1130---."

Kathy was right. Sophia could not believe how many people were here. And on the Upper East Side! she thought as if alcoholics only belonged in the Village.

John was the moderator tonight and he asked Patrick, the man who had been sharing his story since Sophia arrived, to stop for the minute before midnight so everyone could listen to the bells count down the seconds to the new year.

"May we all have a sober one. Happy 1993," John said when the chiming stopped.

Patrick continued to tell the smoke-filled room about the Christmas work dinner he had to attend with all of the other salesmen. He kept one vodka tonic on the table, within reach the whole night, so it looked like he was socializing. He never took a sip.

Everyone clapped. He sat down.

Seats in the second last row opened up. People were leaving who felt safe enough now to venture back out into the world after experiencing a dry ringing in of the year.

Sophia sat down and lit a cigarette. A young woman walked up to the podium and started to talk. She could have been 21 or 31 years old. It was hard to tell because she already looked world-worn.

Everyone said, "Hi, Yvonne" after she introduced herself. Then she began, at her beginning.

Yvonne had not had a drink since her last blackout landed her coatless and purseless in the Bowery. That was this past February. When she came to, she could not feel her body. The temperature had dropped to 5 degrees that night before the wind chill was factored in. She managed to crawl her way to The Village Community Center's ER where she was treated for hypothermia and lost only one toe to frostbite.

Was she really one of these people? Sophia felt nervous again. What could she say that they hadn't heard before? Did she really have that much of a drinking problem?

The moderator asked if anyone new to the group tonight would like to share a story.

Sophia stood up and took a deep breath. "Hi, everyone. I'm Sophia. I'm an alcoholic."

"Hi, Sophia."

She walked to the podium. "At least I think I am."

She began. "I never really cared for the taste of alcohol. When I turned 17 my mother, like any good Italian mother, served me one glass of wine when we had big family dinners. I usually only had a sip or two, just to be polite.

"In nursing school, I only drank at parties and I didn't go to many of them, except when I had a big exam coming up. I would get so nervous about family, about letting them down if I didn't make it through.

"One Saturday night before my big Anatomy and Physiology final, one Jack and Coke led to seven. I wasn't nervous then.

"I had all day Sunday to clear my head for the test. By the time my nerves kicked back in, it was Monday morning. I did fine on the exam.

"So that's sort of how it has gone for me ever since. But it all seems to be speeding up now."

Everyone clapped. She went back to her seat. She felt a little bit of relief. She lit a cigarette.

It was 3 A.M. now but Sophia felt wide awake, even more so than usual, even when on duty.

A man around her age walked towards her as she waited for the crowd to thin its way out the door.

"I'm Ricky. Ricky Abbott. You did a great job, especially for a newbie. You're real honest. That's what helps the most. I think so anyway."

"How long have you been coming here?" Sophia asked.

"Long enough, but not too long that I don't need the security of being with others tonight like me, drunks not drinking on New Year's Eve."

She laughed a little and thought he had a southern accent.

"Would you like to get a "good" cup of coffee? I know a

place on 84th that serves the best all night long. And they have grits and gravy with the best dang biscuits you'll ever have north of the Mason Dixon."

"That sounds good. Hey, where are you from, Ricky?"

"Clinton, North Carolina. My daddy has a pig farm there."

NEW YEAR'S DAY, 1993
Boulevard Diner, 84th and 3rd Avenue, New York City

When the brightness hovering above the street outside rose to Sophia and Ricky's eye level, as Sophia continued to sip her hot chocolate in an effort to wind down for the sleep she needed for her shift tonight, they said they should continue their conversation over another cup of coffee sometime soon.

Hours ago, Sophia had asked Ricky how he made it up here, to the Big Apple. She had only been as far south as Richmond, she told him, and even that was a little too far for her. He told her about where he was raised, in Wilmington, North Carolina, a coastal town on a big river.

"Yet," he said, "I couldn't wait to get the hell out of there. I needed more. Always more."

Ricky did his undergraduate in North Carolina. He could not pass up the scholarship. But when he graduated in 1984, he only had eyes for New York City law schools.

"What made you want to be a lawyer, Ricky?" Sophia asked during their second cup of coffee and second pack of shared Marlboro lights. "By the way, I love the grits," she added.

"I felt like I needed to give a voice to the people who didn't have one, like the homeless everyone walked by or over back home. It's like they were invisible to those standing upright, but they had parents just like me and you, and jobs once."

Sophia was still trying to wrap her head around homeless people living outside of New York City.

"Tell me about you, Sophia. I talk all dang day and here I am doing it again."

"You know I'm from New York, right?"

"I knew for sure when you said you've never had grits before."

Sophia told him about her family in the Bronx. Her parents insisted they lived in Mount Vernon and technically they did on West 1st and 14th Avenue, right over the Bronx line.

She explained her parents were first generation, her mother's parents were from Italy and her father's parents were from Puerto Rico. That meant in order to "have made it" they needed to move out of the Bronx. It also meant their children needed to go to college.

Sophia's older brother, Diego, had no love for books, but he sure could rebuild a car engine. He became a mechanic, a very good one, and he had his own shop on Mount Vernon Avenue, securely out of the Bronx. Diego and his wife, Giada, who Sophia considered a sister, gave her parents two grandchildren, Maria and Mario.

Sophia told Ricky when Diego moved out the pressure fell to her to attend college. Sophia knew she always wanted to be a nurse, ever since she watched her grandmother die from ovarian cancer when she was 14 years old. The nurses always made her grandmother feel better with the tucking in of her favorite blanket, and the conversations they engaged her in about her childhood in Arezzo.

Her parents were thrilled with her career choice but not with her decision to attend a three-year hospital diploma program instead of a four-year college.

"Ma, I want to be an old-fashioned nurse with hands on the first day. My program's three years with no summers off. No slacking there. I can always get a degree later," she repeated the conversation for Ricky.

Her younger sister, Terri, on the other hand got a degree in Art History from a private college in Connecticut. She loved her job as a docent at *The Met* in the Egyptian collection. There wasn't a column built before 300 BCE that Terri couldn't date, she told him; plus, Terri could really draw. But she did not make enough money to move out of her parents' home.

"So, my parents brag about me the most because I 'almost went to college,' as they put it, and I can afford to live on my own in Manhattan. Barely, of course, without doing double shifts in order to go out to dinner whenever I want."

Ricky said his parents were happy with his career choice also, but not with the type of law he chose to practice. "As my mother says, 'all those good schools and no money to show for it. Funny how your brother Bobby earns more without a college degree, just making those cars shiny as they can be'." Ricky said his brother owned his own body shop outside of Wilmington.

"What kind of law do you practice, Ricky?"

"This is really what my mother gets right quiet about." He explained that he trained as a civil rights attorney and was with the CLO, the Civil Liberties Organization, for the first few years out of law school here in New York. But when his old roommate, Steve, got AIDS, a Wall Street lawyer, "like I should have been," Ricky repeated what his mother always said, he left the CLO.

"Is Steve dead?" Sophia asked.

"No sugar coating it, huh, Sophia. Yes. He died last year, but before he did he lost everything when his boss and his land-lord found out about his disease."

"It's disgusting to be treated like that," Sophia said.

"I helped him out as much as I could, volunteered for the

legal team of GCAS. When Steve passed, I joined them full time for even less money than I made at the CLO. Do you know the organization, Sophia?"

"Yes. Very well. The Gay Coalition for AIDS Support has provided some of the only resources my patients receive."

"You work with AIDS patients, Sophia?"

Sophia told him about how she had been an ER nurse for about a year or so, after she graduated from nursing school, at The Upper East Side Medical Center. But she couldn't take how they were treated in the ER, and knew it must have been even worse after they were admitted.

"One night, I finally made it back around to José who had been waiting all day for a bed upstairs in the respiratory unit. He had *PCP*. He was lying in a pool of urine when I checked him. I asked him when he was changed last."

'Nurse. You're the only one who's been in here.'"

That had been six hours earlier, Sophia explained to Ricky. The two trays of food left on the floor outside of José's room, feeding only the roaches Sophia had discovered when she lifted the plate covers, were the measurement of how much time had passed.

"When the AIDS Unit opened in October of 1987, I asked for a transfer. I've been there ever since."

"That's hard core, Sophia."

"Any man I've felt comfortable enough with to even talk about my nursing specialty usually asks for the check at this point. And then politely excuses himself."

Ricky waved to the waiter, and asked for Sophia's phone number

"That pig don't look right, Sam," Reba Smith said standing at the kitchen window looking out at the penned yard in front of the barn.

"He's just fine, Rebe. I'll takes care of 'em later."

"He sure don't look good enough to eat on Christmas, Sam. I thought you got 'em from the best pig farmer up there in Carolina. Maybe that there other one you sold to Bart for pennies is faring better than ours," Reba said.

"He just needs some more soy bean, Rebe. That's all. I'll gets some this afternoon."

Sam Smith had no intention of feeding this piglet, now 11 weeks old. When he brought the little guy home from Porky's Farm at Halloween, he led his wife to believe it would be for Christmas dinner, just as he thought he led her to believe that he joined a charity for albino blind children where the members wore white hoods so they could understand how it felt not to see.

Reba Smith knew she better make her way to the big market in Birmingham if she had any chance of finding a decent Christmas ham.

"I'll be back in a few, Sam."

Sam knew she meant hours, not minutes.

Sam stood in the doorway watching Reba drive away. Then he walked over to the barn and waited.

There were ten of them now standing inside the barn with the door shut. The piglet was in the middle of all of the men with their heads covered.

Sam began. "We's gathered here to honor all those little babes being killed by thems wicked mothers in the devil's clinics in Birmingham."

"Amen," replied the others.

"We need to keep 'em alive so ours race don't die."

"Amen."

Sam Smith removed his hood and the other men did the same. Two of them held the slippery little animal, struggling with all his limited might to get free, while Sam raised the axe.

The head fell to the ground. Another man placed the big jar under the piglet's neck and collected the blood pouring out while two of the others continued to hold the body.

When the piglet stopped moving and the blood stopped flowing, the men let the little carcass fall to the ground. They only noticed now that the pig's body was covered in purplish blotches.

"What in hell's name is that there?" one of them said pointing to the discoloration as he kicked the carcass aside.

Sam placed the big jar filled with the pig's blood in the center of the men and said, "Here's to President Jefferson Davis. May we keep the South alive. May we keep them white babies alive. We be sure to put an end to them clinics soon."

And then they dipped their fingers in the bowl and painted crosses on each other's foreheads all the while trying to stop the blood from dripping into their eyes.

DECEMBER 24, 2020
Florence, Italy

St. Sebastian's church bells were ringing for hours in the piazza. Sophia embraced Ricky through their echo. She remembered they, especially Ricky, could not resist buying this apartment during their 10th anniversary trip in 2005.

"Come now," Sophia. We can afford it."

"I hope so. It is beautiful," Sophia said to Ricky as they

walked around the living room while Ricky inspected the walls for any signs of disrepair.

"We'll pay for it all. In cash."

"Yes, but Ricky, what about the taxes? And the utilities?"

"There's more than enough left over, darling, after all these years of me working for them richies. It'll be our reward," he said.

Ricky kissed her when they reached the large mullioned window opening out over the stone-lined Via San Gallo Street two stories below.

A few years ago, Sophia felt like she had no choice but to move here into this nineteenth century one bedroom apartment with a comfy-sized living space, working kitchen, and one bathroom just blocks from the *Academy* where she popped in almost daily to admire Michelangelo's masterpiece. She felt close to Ricky when she stood at the feet of the statue with a tinge of worry in his eyes.

AUGUST, 2017
New York City

The #6 down to 14th Street stopped dead in its tracks at 33rd for about 20 minutes. Not an unusual occurrence but not a good one today when Sophia needed to meet with Darcy, a 16 year-old-girl who was trying to shake her addiction to Oxycodone when her pregnancy test turned positive.

Sophia had been working as a counselor at the Lower East Side Women's Center for almost 20 years now. All the classes she had been taking while working on the AIDS Unit at The Upper East Side Medical Center gave her enough credits to complete a degree in psychology by 1995, just in time for the revolution in AIDS treatment: HAART (Highly Active Anti-retroviral Therapy).

Sophia never could have imagined that a few more anti-retrovirals added to the AZT she had given to patients for years, as she watched them feel even worse after taking it, would raise them from their sick beds and release them back into the world to dine out, shop, and even work again.

When the hospital administrators started talking about filling the empty beds with oncology patients, Sophia knew it was time to leave. Cancer patients died more often than not in 1995 with the age of immunotherapy still years away. And she did not have it in her to carry on with another hopeless patient population now that the AIDS wave was crashing on the shores of life.

Ricky's caseload at GCAS had lightened in conjunction with Sophia's beds emptying. He was making enough for the two of them after they married, right as she left hospital nursing. He had taken on discrimination cases for old money 5th Avenue denizens who were now suing the hell out of doctors, hospitals, and school boards who provided less than adequate services to their family members who got AIDS in the late 1980s or early 1990s and lived, just long enough, to receive the life-saving drugs.

Sophia started studying full time for her Masters in Social Work after she and Ricky returned from their honeymoon in Italy. She became an addictions counselor and, not surprisingly, was very good at it.

When Sophia took any patients to their first meeting, she would always stand up before they did and introduce herself as an alcoholic. That surprised them, but they trusted her even more.

She had been counseling Darcy throughout this summer. The young girl had been clean for eight weeks, but now had to decide what to do about being pregnant. Darcy said she "felt too fucked up" to have a baby now. She was almost 12 weeks along and she knew the placental blood inside her womb was rich with Oxycodone the first 4 weeks of her pregnancy. The doctor had warned her that damage could have been done to the baby during that time.

Sophia walked Darcy through her decision. Could she live with terminating her pregnancy? How would she feel at 30? Would she regret an abortion? What were her goals after high school? She was smart, Sophia knew that after a few sessions, and she wanted to study environmental law. Would a baby at this age make her goals just a dream, or would taking care of a little human keep her committed to a drug-free life and a good career?

The problem now, Sophia knew all too well, since President Rumpel and his party won the White House and both chambers of Congress in the last election, was how to find an experienced doctor who would still perform the abortion Darcy decided to have in the end.

Bills had been moving through so many state legislatures trying to restrict and even overturn the federal law that made abortion legal way back in the early 1970s. Sophia could not believe the country her grandparents traveled to from the Tuscan mountains in Italy and the streets of San Juan, Puerto Rico, dreaming of a life filled with freedoms and opportunities, wanted to return women to the mercy of back alley butchers.

No state had overturned the federal law yet, but it was coming. OB/GYN doctors who had performed abortions for years were getting nervous, even in states like New York that were not considering restrictions yet. And many of the doctors feared the federal government might retroactively hold them accountable as "murderers," if they performed the procedure after the 12th week of pregnancy.

Sophia sent emails to all the local papers. She posted on medical blogs for women's health issues. She said experienced doctors were needed to perform safe abortions, especially for a young girl nearing her 13th week of pregnancy now. She asked where she could send her patient.

Sophia thought she would get a few responses to her pleas. Instead, one evening she received a knock on her and Ricky's brownstone door on 88th and York Avenue, the bargain that fell into her lap after they returned from their honeymoon in 1995.

One of Sophia's patients, Ed, wrote a letter to her after she left the unit. Sura, a fellow night shift nurse for years, made sure Sophia got it after Ed died from a cryptococcal infection in his bowels and brain. Ed told them, "At least I still *know* when I have to shit my brains out, but what happens when I actually do? I hope I'm gone by then."

Ed had stated in his will that he wanted his "niece," Sophia, to move into his rent-controlled apartment when he died. His rent was fixed at $300 per month since 1968 when he acquired it from his great Aunt Emily.

On the other side of the door, when Sophia opened it, letting the dirty, humid air in, stood a squirrely-looking man with a subpoena for Sophia to appear in court for offensive language used in her recent emails.

"What are you talking about, sir? I haven't said anything the least bit offensive to anyone since our last election night when that man carrying a Rumpel sign told me I didn't look American enough to vote."

"I've been told, Ms. Lorenzo, or is it Mrs. Abbott? You are married to one Richard Abbott, aren't you?"

"My name is Sophia Maria Lorenzo. And yes, I have been married to Richard Abbott for a long time now, but he's been dead for the last nine years of it."

"I'm sorry Ms. Lorenzo. I have to issue you this subpoena to appear in court. The current administration has developed new standards of speech to be used in public. You will need to be in US District Court on September 21, 2017 at 9 A.M.," he said, and then handed her the papers.

Sophia slammed the door shut and fell onto her couch. "What the hell's going on?"

OCTOBER 10, 2017
Midtown Public Library, New York City

The court ordered Sophia to attend "speech therapy classes" so she could learn "how to appropriately discuss sensitive public issues." Classes started tonight and would be held every Tuesday from 7 to 9 P.M. for six weeks.

She loved this library, but the more she thought about what she had to do, the more nauseated she became walking through the reading room with its dark wooded walls and long tables harboring green lights brightening just the right spot on every one of them.

Sophia still could not believe Alvin Rumpel got elected last November. He had no experience in politics or public service, unless the big restaurant chain he owned where his workers had no health insurance and barely earned minimum wage qualified. He really only had even that thanks to his father who had been a Chicago steel magnate.

But Rumpel made promises to all the people who could no longer make decent livings in manufacturing jobs, such as the steel and automobile industries. There were enough of them who believed in him, plus the electoral college was bound to vote for his party in most of the districts of every state drawn in his favor.

Sophia found the classroom. It was the only light she could

see in the long hallway on the other side of the reading room. When she sat down she noticed all of the students' faces were brown like hers, or darker. The instructor was unpacking his bag on the table in the front of the room. He looked pissed off and uncomfortable. His face was not so brown.

He placed a government-issued book on everyone's desk, *Language for a Better America*, while explaining the purpose of this class. Public spaces had become cesspools for unpatriotic language and people needed to speak more respectfully about our country.

For the next six weeks, each student would read a piece of writing by someone else in the class and grow to understand what was anti-American in it. By the end of the class, each student would be able to use language that honored the values and ideals of the republic once again.

Sophia wanted to shout. She wanted to run out into the streets. But this was court-ordered indoctrination. She could not risk arrest or anything else that might prevent her from what she now knew she needed to do.

LATE DECEMBER, 2017
New York City

Sophia had given her four weeks' notice at the Lower East Side Women's Center during Halloween week after almost 20 years of service. Her boss, Ella, was concerned she could find another counselor with the compassion and passion Sophia brought to her role. Her colleagues and patients were saddened by the news.

The speech therapy classes ended two days before Thanksgiving. Sophia applied for her entrance visa at the Italian consulate that week. It would allow her to live in Italy for at least 90 days. They assured her it would be ready within two weeks. So she bought a plane ticket, one way to Rome, with a connecting train to Florence for December 20th.

Thankfully, she did not have to contend with moving out of the brownstone. One of her sister's colleagues at the museum needed an apartment fast and Sophia was all too happy to sublet hers for at least three years, or as long as it took for this country to begin veering off the dangerous path it had taken.

Terri's colleague was thrilled to pay $700 more per month than what Sophia paid because it was still $1000 less than the small studio she was losing on the Upper West Side.

That left Sophia's clothing and favorite books to pack for her move, and checking on the status of her visa daily. She thought she would be able to visit her father-in-law in North Carolina before she left but she had to settle for calling him instead.

She told Tucker Abbott she was moving to Florence. She told him he needed to visit, for as long as he liked, and he should do some sightseeing in Europe, as well.

"I know, Sophia. Ricky always told me that too when the two of you bought the place. But now that Emma's gone, I don't care too much about getting away from the farm."

Ricky's mother, Emma, had died from ovarian cancer, just like Sophia's grandmother did so many years ago. Sophia nursed her through the intense pain in her basketball sized abdomen. Ovarian cancer still looked pretty much like it did in the 1970s, Sophia thought, when she lifted up Emma's stick-like limbs during the final baths she gave her in 2012. She sure was glad she did not stay on the AIDS Unit in 1995 when it transitioned to oncology.

"I know you miss her, Tucker. I do too," Sophia told her father-in-law during this last conversation before she left the country.

"I'll miss seeing you, darl'n. I always enjoy your Christmas visits."

"Me too, Tucker."

"I'll tell you what though, Sophia. If I were a woman in this here country today and was able to go elsewhere, I'd go. It's all go'n to hell in a handbasket. That new law they're trying to pass for women filing for divorce hav'n to prove with pictures that their husbands beat them or messed around on them is just too much, even for me."

Sophia was a bit surprised Tucker Abbott felt this way because he always erred on the conservative side in politics. But she also knew he always respected women a great deal.

"Love you, Tuck."

"Me too. You be safe now. Don't walk out on your own at night. I know it's Florence but there's bound to be hoodlums. They're everywhere."

She was home now. She always called it that even though she hadn't lived there in over 30 years. Mrs. Lorenzo had burst into tears when Sophia told her about her decision to leave America during Thanksgiving dinner.

"Hey, Ma. It's me," she yelled when she walked in the front door.

"I'm in the kitchen. Coffee's almost ready."

She kissed her mother on the cheek at the sink where she was standing.

"Will you be back?"

"I will be back to visit, for sure, if the government still allows its citizens living abroad to return."

"You have a passport, Sophia."

"I used to be able to say what I wanted to say also."

"I must admit, I thought it was just you at first, Sophia, blowing things out of proportion, like you do. But Mrs. Torrea next door is 90 now and loves the internet. Gets around on it better than me. She always says when I see her pick a tomato from her garden, 'Getting ready to go surfing.'

"Anyway, she wrote an email to our congressman telling him she wasn't happy they moved her voting poll to the Bronx River Parkway instead of keeping it down the street at St. Paul's Grade School where she has been voting for years. She wrote how it would take her two buses and a good amount of walking to get there.

"Next thing you know, she's subpoenaed, like you were for these speech therapy classes."

"It's getting scary, Ma. Do you want to come with me?"

"You know I can't. I have the grandchildren."

"Diego and Giada's are grown, Ma, and don't even live in New York."

"I have June."

"I know, and she adores you. Are you over the fact me and Ricky didn't give you any?"

"You have your children, Sophia. You always have."

"Oh, let me update you on my patient, Darcy, the one I tried to find a doctor for in order to perform the ..."

"Don't say it, Sophia," Mrs. Lorenzo held up her hand to interrupt her daughter.

"OK, Ma. I respect your beliefs but just listen."

Mrs. Lorenzo was still standing by the sink looking at the floor.

"I never could find anyone. So, Darcy's last ultrasound, the one she had right before I resigned, in her second trimester, showed the baby had anencephaly."

Mrs. Lorenzo's raised her head with her eyes widening.

"Her baby had only half a head, thanks to the Oxy she was still taking during the first four weeks when she didn't even know she was pregnant."

"Now what, Sophia? My God."

"She will either miscarry or deliver the baby at full term. Either way, it cannot live."

. They sat down at the table. Mrs. Lorenzo had bought a beautiful panettone from her favorite bakery, Alfonso's, on Arthur Avenue in the Bronx. They were waiting for Diego and Giada. Sophia's niece, Maria, lived in Philadelphia now and worked in pharmaceuticals, and her nephew, Mario, did something in finance up in Boston.

Mrs. Lorenzo sat at the table in silence for a few minutes and then said, "It should be allowed in cases like hers. That poor girl."

"That's what's so wrong, Ma. Our rights are withering away. And there's talk now that Rumpel is going to sign a law to ban gay marriage again."

The president's executive orders could now bypass the House and go right to the Senate to become law if national security threats were the subject. His wily lawyers crafted the rationale for banning gay marriage: If natural reproduction cannot occur in a marriage, then the American population will decline in number and in kind. If that happens, our military might will weaken.

"What will happen to Terri and Leslie and my darling June?" Mrs. Lorenzo was starting to panic.

Terri had married Leslie two years ago, right after Mr. Lorenzo died from his third stroke. Terri had introduced Leslie to her family, a guard at the museum, as her good friend about five years ago.

Mrs. Lorenzo knew. She knew ever since Tony Leote, the most handsome boy in her high school, asked Terri to the prom and she refused to go. Terri never went with any boys then or since.

Mrs. Lorenzo grew to care for Leslie, love her, especially

after Terri gave birth to June, the product of artificial insemination after they married.

Diego and Giada arrived. They stopped talking about gay marriage. Diego could barely tolerate Terri and Leslie's relationship let alone acknowledge their marriage. And he certainly could not understand why Sophia was moving to Italy.

"What'd ya thinks gonna happen to you here, Soph? I mean they're not gonna lock you up for speak'n you're mind, heh. It's not like you've threatened to kill anyone," he said to her after they kissed hello.

"Well, bro, I was sentenced to take classes so I don't say what I want to say in an email ever again."

"Maybe you're just too sensitive. All those years tak'n care of them freaks makes you think the world's still 'gainst you.

"And look at 'em now. They marry for Christ's sake and get all them drugs for free to keep 'em alive forever."

"Well, that's not quite accurate. And your own sister, Diego, is one of them so-called freaks. She's with the person she loves. Why do you care anyway about who somebody loves?"

"That's what I try an tell 'em, Soph," Giada chimed in.

"I don't wanna hear anything out of you, Giad. It's bad enough two women in my family don't know their place. Not you too," Diego said.

Sophia knew at this point there was no sense in responding anymore to her brother's idiocy. So she asked about their children instead.

After Giada drank a cup of coffee and had a slice of the Italian sweet bread and Diego drank two beers, they started to say goodbye.

"I wish I could come with," Giada whispered in Sophia's ear as they hugged each other.

"Any problems, you call, Soph. I'll be there in a New York

minute to rough 'em up," Diego said as he kissed her on each cheek.

"Will you see your sister before you leave, Sophia?" Mrs. Lorenzo asked as the front door closed.

"Tomorrow night I'm meeting them for dinner at the new French restaurant that's all the rave on the Upper West Side."

"I love you, Sophia. You always have a home. Call me when you can, but always on Sundays at least."

"Love you, Mom," she said as she hugged her mother knowing it would be a long time until she did again.

December 24, 2020
Florence, Italy

The pasteles were almost ready. Instead of stuffing the tamale-like Christmas recipe with pork, handed down from her father's side of the family, Sophia filled them with finely diced prawns, from the Italian side.

She was going over to Kat and Luigi's for a quiet celebration before going to midnight mass at Il Duomo, inside the Cathedral of Santa Maria there. Sophia met Kat, a nurse, at the English Women's Clinic where she started working as a counselor about a year ago after she established her permanent residency in Florence and completed all of the requirements for mastering Italian language, culture, and civics.

Most of the expatriate nurses, doctors, counselors, and administrative staff at the clinic had run away from their own countries, and flocked to Florence waiting for the next great renaissance.

Sophia could not believe it had been three years since she moved here, but felt like she still could not return with abortion only allowed now in the States before six weeks of gestation

and gay marriage definitively illegal once again. And then Terri
had written to her about the conversion centers that were
popping up for transgender people.

These issues, and many more, were hot topics of conversation tonight at the Christmas Eve dinner she attended. Kat was
British but it was her husband Luigi who talked the most about
why they fled England last year.

His engineering firm, based in Rome, had opened an office
in London a few years ago and he jumped at the chance to
work in it. He fell in love with British routines, mannerisms,
tea, and Kat. But last year the new Prime Minister started
imposing a residency tax of 6,000 pounds per annum on
anyone who was not born in England.

Even though Luigi had married Kat, born in Richmond,
outside of London, he still had to pay. Luigi felt like it was the
sign of much worst things to come. They moved to Florence
last year when a position opened up in his firm here. And they
were really pleased they did because the British government
now was asking all non-natives to leave the country before the
ban on immigrants became law.

As the small group discussed these problems, they had the
comfort of a few bottles of Barolo, a bottle of sparkling water for
Sophia, and the scrumptious dishes served. Luigi made gnocchi
with three cheeses in pesto sauce and Sophia's pasteles were a
good compliment. Their friend Barbara from Wisconsin made
irresistible pierogies, her Polish family's old recipe of potato
dumplings sautéed in onions. Kat topped it all off nicely with
some classic plum pudding and a pot of Earl Grey tea.

At 11 P.M. they walked the few blocks to the church. They
wanted to get there early so some seats could be had for mass.
Sophia loved it in here at Christmas time with the floor to
ceiling trees in the cathedral's transept and the golden lights
adorning the arches.

When her friends found their spots, Sophia walked around the trees some more and then snuck back to her Via San Gallo apartment. Sophia always loved the architectural beauty of Europe's churches, especially Italy's, thanks to her sister's private lessons whenever they toured together, but she had not gotten much at all from the Catholic religion, or any other, since her second year of work on the AIDS Unit in 1988.

She called her father-in-law when she reached the apartment. She knew it was still early enough in North Carolina.

"Buon Natale, Tucker," Sophia said when he answered his wall phone with the long cord. He was the only person she knew who did not have some sort of mobile phone.

"Sophia? How are you? What time is it there?" he always asked her that expecting to hear it was North Carolina time.

"I'm fine, Tucker. It's going on midnight."

"Aren't you Italians supposed to be in church right about now?"

"Well, I was. But I wanted to talk to some family instead. I guess you're not doing much of anything tonight, Tucker?"

"Not tonight, darl'n. You sure must miss your family's big shindig back in New York."

"It's not nearly as big now, Tucker, with my father dead and so many aunts and uncles gone, too. I tell you what, though, I'll never forget the first Christmas Eve I brought Ricky home. Everyone was alive and well then."

CHRISTMAS EVE, 1993
Mount Vernon, New York

Sophia's parents liked Ricky Abbott right from the start, even her father.

"A lawyer, hmm," Mr. Lorenzo said after they walked into

the house swelling with people in every room, including the kitchen.

"Nice to meet you, sir," Ricky said as he handed him a bottle of Bacardi Rum with a velvet red ribbon tied around the neck.

"Thank you very much. Sophia tells me you help the gays like she does."

"Well not everyone with AIDS is gay, Mr. Lorenzo."

"Yeah, I know, Ricky, but there's a lot of that going around. I mean being gay. My daughter Terri tells me she is now, too."

"Terri's a good one, just like Sophia. She designs GCAS posters and we've gotten lots of donations because of them. And what she charges can't be beat. She does it for free."

"How would you like a drink, Ricky? Some of that good rum you got me with some coke."

"Just a coke would be great, Mr. Lorenzo."

"Call me, Juan."

Ricky charmed more than Sophia's father that evening. Her mother and aunts thought he was so polite, well-spoken, and even handsome, 'in spite of how pale-looking he was,' Aunt Sylvia said. And all of the women loved to hear him talk.

After about two hours, Sophia thought Ricky needed some rescuing. She knew he was not accustomed to all the hugs and kisses he received with every introduction. Sophia told her mom they had promised one of Ricky's friends on the Upper East Side that they would stop in for some egg nog before the night was over.

After another half an hour of good bye hugs and kisses and plenty of invitations to First Communions and graduations, they were outside in the crisp night.

"Sophia, we could have stayed longer."

"That was a lot. I know."

"They made me feel real welcome. I hope my family does

28

the same with you. You won't get all that affection. But if my mom allows you to help with the cooking, and she will, you're in."

CHRISTMAS EVE, 2020
Florence, Italy

Tucker told Sophia he would drive to Bobby and Sue Ellen's tomorrow, Ricky's younger brother and his wife who lived about an hour away. Their four grown children would be there to celebrate the holiday, as well, with their own families.

"I hope I can eat alright though," Tucker said on the other end of the phone.

"Have you not been feeling well? You should have called, Tucker."

"Well, hell. No big deal. My bowels have seen better days. I had a real friendly relationship with my toilet between Halloween and Thanksgiving. Less familiar since."

"Did you see a doctor?"

"No, cause it's much better. I just need to be careful with the food."

"It sounds like you might have had a virus, Tucker. It still wouldn't hurt to see a doctor."

"Merry Christmas, Sophia. Talk to you soon."

FEBRUARY 9, 2021
Savannah, Georgia

The heat snuck into this port city earlier and earlier every year, forcing the Spanish moss in Forsyth Park to carry its moisture longer and longer. Robin Wake was cycling through the park at

6:30 A.M. Her scrub top was wet when she parked her bike outside of one of the oldest hospitals in the United States.

"How y'all?" she said to the nurses, preparing for shift report, walking past the station.

"Hey, Dr. Wake," a night nurse said.

"Hey, Robin," Sally, a day shift nurse said.

Dr. Winston Taylor started telling her all about the night as she changed her top in the bathroom of the on-call room.

"If it wasn't bad enough that a 22-year old woman came in with a gunshot wound to her lower back after her two-year old son found her gun and started playing with it."

"Was she admitted?"

"Thankfully, the bullet just grazed her skin. She only needed a few stitches. I discharged her about an hour ago.

"But last evening we got this transfer from down in Darien," Winston continued.

He explained to Robin that the community hospital in Darien, a small port town about an hour south of Savannah, was not equipped to provide higher level medical care for this 45-year-old male who had been admitted there this past weekend.

That hospital, though, was able to find a pharmacy that still carried Diluted Tincture of Opium (DTO), the only drug slowing down Mr. George Johnson's copious diarrhea. Winston had never even heard of the brown drops of stool-stopping magic when the much older Darien doctor gave him the patient's history over the phone.

Mr. Johnson's diarrhea, the doctor told Winston, was now 10 times per day, whereas before the DTO was given every two hours, it had been 25, plus the patient's weight had dropped by 12 pounds in just three days. All of the stool cultures were negative, which meant there was no sense in prescribing any antibiotics.

Then Winston told Robin how somber the Darien doctor got when he reported Mr. Johnson's temperature spike to 103 degrees Fahrenheit accompanied by a new, wet cough. The chest x-ray showed pneumonia but the Azithromycin they gave the patient for the past 48 hours did not help his symptoms at all. This patient clearly needed a bigger hospital and a better diagnosis.

Robin responded. "I don't know about you, Winston, but my infectious disease rotation did not show me anything too, too serious. All of the older doctors told us about the days of exotic plague-like infections in AIDS patients before the era of antiretrovirals. Heck, even when I did a month's rotation in an HIV clinic in Atlanta, I only saw one case of PCP and that was because the young man hadn't been taking his meds."

"I saw more than that, Robin, during my training in North Carolina, but I don't think this patient from Darien has it. And ID thought the same last night," Winston said.

"When did Infectious Diseases see him?" Robin asked.

"Right after he arrived. They ordered a whole bunch of blood, sputum, and urine tests, including HIV. We're waiting on a bed for him up on pulmonary."

"He's in isolation, right?"

"Hell, yeah. We're not taking any chances with TB. It's probably not, but we need to see."

By noon that day a bed opened up for Mr. Johnson. Sally Jenkins, RN, took over his care around 10 A.M. and she had some of the results to review with Dr. Wake.

"Hi, Sally," Robin said when the nurse caught her ready to see another patient behind closed curtains. "I thought Melba had Johnson today."

"Well she did, but the patient kept shaking his head no when she tried to check his IV or hang an antibiotic or even fix his sheets a little."

"That's weird."

"Not really. His wife told me, after Melba asked me to take care of him, that he prefers only people 'like him' to touch him."

"What does that mean?"

"I think she meant only white people."

"Damn. How pathetic is that. So, what do you have, Sally?"

"It looks like Johnson has *Mycoplasma* pneumonia."

"Well at least we know now what antibiotics will work."

"HIV?

"No HIV," the nurse said.

"It couldn't be that easy, could it?" the doctor said.

"No, but listen to this." Sally went on to tell Robin a little more about the night shift nurse's report. She had been in Mr. Johnson's room when the ID doctor tried to find out more information about the patient's exposure to any viruses, bacteria, or even parasites.

The doctor asked Mrs. Johnson if her husband had been out of the country in the last six months or near anyone who had been.

"He sure ain't been anywhere outside of our one donkey town until last night when Georgie was transferred here. I ain't been to Savannah since I was a little girl. Anyway, the only place George's been is that pig farm up in North Carolina."

Then the night nurse said Mrs. Johnson explained that her husband was with some of his friends from up in Atlanta and someone named Sam from Alabama. They all travelled to Clinton, North Carolina at Halloween time to buy some piglets so some blind children could have some Christmas dinners. Mrs. Johnson said those fellas all belonged to some charity.

Then the night nurse quoted what Mrs. Johnson said next about the piglets.

"All them spent a pretty penny on them but that didn't matter no how. The one in our pen couldn't barely stand up by

Thanksgiving. And he looked a little purplish all over. Georgie had to shoot the little thing, back of the barn, first weekend in December. That's what he told me."

Near the end of her 12-hour shift, Dr. Robin Wake received a call from a clinic near Darien. They had three patients who needed ambulance transfer to Savannah General. All of the men were middle aged with diarrhea for about a week and now with high fevers and wicked coughs.

SAN VALENTINO, 2021
Florence, Italy

Sophia lit the one candle sitting on the table set for two. She did every year for Ricky.

SAN VALENTINO, 2007
Florence, Italy

They decided to have a little getaway at their Florentine apartment about a week ago. Ricky had been feeling tired and Sophia thought he was putting in too many hours at the CLO where he returned after they bought this place a few years ago.

Ricky felt like he still had a lot of wrongs to right, especially for browns and Blacks who always ended up with heavy court fines and jail time in comparison to white criminals.

Sophia had been looking forward to some time away from the Women's Center. She had been counseling Louisa, a young Mexican woman who just found out she was HIV positive, but really had full blown AIDS already. Her viral load was super high and her T cells were super low, which meant, as Sophia knew all too well, she would be very ill if antiretrovirals were not started immediately.

But Louisa did not want to take any medications. What would Manny think? Her boyfriend already had such a bad temper when he could not get his "medicine," that's what he liked to call the heroin he needed more than once a day now.

Sophia's concern was getting Louisa to think about her own health and guiding her towards acceptance of taking the medicine that would save her life.

Ricky had planned one of the most romantic Valentine's Days ever. They would begin the morning at their favorite café for espressos and sfratti, those heavenly honey walnut cookie sticks, and then walk it off on their way to the *Uffizi*. Lunch would be perfect at the trattoria near the *Academy* with zucchini and mozzarella stuffed bread baked just right. The *Academy* would top off the day before the chef Ricky hired to make an antipasto platter followed by shrimp scampi and then Bolognese papparedella arrived at their Via San Gallo apartment.

But at the *Academy*, standing together holding hands, admiring *David*, Sophia noticed something different when she looked at Ricky. Maybe it was just the lighting. Ricky's skin looked a little orange, like the flavored seltzer drink they had at lunch, and his eyes looked a little yellow.

She kept this observation to herself, not wanting to ruin this perfect day or to alarm her husband. She always tended to be hopeless about any medical problems experienced by anyone she loved.

San Valentino, 2021
Florence, Italy

Sophia sat at their table in the dining room staring into the flame and remembered every hour of that night, their last Valentine's Day in 2007. But, for the first time now, she would go beyond the wonderful dinner and the lovemaking, and Ricky's protective embrace until the morning sun filled the living room she could see from their bed.

Sophia went to the doctor's diagnosis, starting with the bloodwork she urged Ricky to have when they returned to New York. The hepatitis C results led to a CT scan. And then there it was: Stage IV liver cancer. Why couldn't his damn virus have waited for the cure? she thought.

Tucker and Emma visited Ricky before he was bed bound, regrettably it was their only trip to New York City. But they did get to *Radio City Music Hall* and watched the ice skaters at Rockefeller Center. Emma loved the Rockettes the most.

When hospice came on board, Sophia worked with the nurse as if it was 1989. She knew when Ricky needed a cool cloth and when he needed a warm one for his head. She knew when to drop the liquid morphine under his tongue to make his moans go away, and when to rub the Haldol gel onto his arm to soothe his whimpers.

Ricky had gotten himself out of bed in the evening for the first time in weeks. He spoke forcefully and intelligently as if he were arguing a case in front of his toughest judge. Sophia knew he would not be there the next day. Always the quiet before the storm, always the surge of energy and mental acuity before it all slips away for good.

He asked for a cigarette. They had quit together about a year ago, but she always had an unopened pack in case of an emergency.

"Sophia," he began as he put out the cigarette and took a bite of the brioche from their favorite bakery on York Avenue.

"I couldn't have been any happier in my life. You've given me so much. You are my companion in love, intellect, and recovery."

Sophia felt like she needed a big glass of red wine as Ricky spoke his final soliloquy.

"I am so sorry," Ricky continued.

"For what, Ricky? You have nothing to be sorry for, honey. We've always been honest with ourselves and with each other."

"You remember my friend Steve I told you about from law school?"

"Yes, of course. You told me the first night we met. He died of AIDS. You don't have AIDS, Ricky. You were tested along with the hepatitis."

"I know I don't have AIDS. Just listen, Sophia. Please.

"For a brief period of time, near the end of law school, Steve and I got into coke. Who didn't? It was the '80s. We heard we could really get a good burst of energy if we ...."

"Shot it," Sophia interrupted him.

"Right. We had our review course exams for the bar coming up. We didn't want to actually try it out for the bar itself. We needed all the time we could get to study and sleeping was interfering with it, but if we could just skip sleep.

"Steve went first after the liquid cooled in the spoon and then I used the same needle."

Sophia's response was more clinical than emotional.

"Oh, I see now, Ricky, Steve had hepatitis but not HIV yet, right?"

"Must've been like that otherwise HIV would have been in my blood too."

"I wondered where you picked it up. I just figured it was from sex with someone, even though it's hard to get that way. If anyone should have gotten hepatitis C, it should've been me from some of the sticks I had back then at work."

"I'm glad you didn't get it, Sophia."

"Well, me too in the end. But like I said before, Ricky Abbott, you have nothing to be sorry about. You made a mistake that has hurt you more than you ever should have been hurt."

"I'm just sorry I don't get to grow old with you," Ricky said.

"Me, too," she looked down so he would not see her tears.

Ricky had another cigarette. He looked serene.

Sophia helped him back to bed. He did not need any more morphine or Haldol.

Sometime in the 4 o'clock hour, he went to sleep for good.

February 15, 2021
Florence, Italy

Sophia's dark night of memories led her to think next about what her sister had told her on the phone when they spoke over the holidays. She felt the lid on her Pandora's box starting to open.

CHRISTMAS DAY, 2020
Florence, Italy

"Terri, what are you saying? The president is only going to allow it to be on display this once? How fucking noble of him."

"Calm down, Sophia. We all know he's horrible, reelected I don't know how."

"I do, Terri. People stopped believing that voting even mattered."

"It will be laid out on the National Mall in D.C."

"When is it?"

"June 5--12th."

"At least they got that right," Sophia said.

"You mean the beginning," Terri said.

"Yeah. It'll be 40 years on June 5, 2021. That's when the first case of AIDS was reported by the Central Disease Bureau, the CDB. Does it still exist, Terri?"

"Yeah that does but Rumpel stopped funding to it and to the National Health Centers. There's only one hospital left in Crystal City, Virginia."

"Who's funding the CDB?"

"Some very pissed off Atlantans who got very rich from rap and hip hop back in the day thought it might be a good idea to keep it around. I heard one of them give an interview last year. They don't want people in their community to die again for years before anyone takes notice.

"I also read these musicians have money for the CDB to pay hospitals who report any new diseases."

"Maybe there is hope, Terri."

"Sophia, I know you don't like to talk about it. Those years. But this might be a way to start. Have you ever seen the Quilt. I mean the whole thing?"

"No. I know I need to. I was with many of them as they made their panels, their portable cloth coffins."

"You sure were, Soph. And thank God for you and the others."

Sophia said nothing.

"Guess who I saw in the museum last week? I was walking to the Egyptian room and took a shortcut through one of the temporary exhibits, one on Holocaust artifacts."

"You mean, like jewelry and teeth? How gruesome, Terri. So who?"

"Your old friend, Sura. Sura Weber, right?"

"Talk about a ghost from the past. How is she? I am not surprised she was at that exhibit."

"She looks old. I never realized how many years she had on you, Sophia."

"Well, let's see. I was in my early 20s in the late '80s and she was in her mid-50s, at least. She was ready to retire, I remember, when it hit."

"She remembered me, and Leslie, and I told her about June. And, of course, she asked about you. You two kind of lost touch, she said, after Ricky died in 2008."

"I lost touch with a lot then, as you know, Ter."

"Sura was with Liz. I thought she had a husband, but Liz sure did look like a wife. Not that we can say that now."

"She must've lost Harold, her husband. He was a sweetheart. He shared her with Liz. That's the kind of man he was. He loved Sura deeply."

"They will be there, Sophia, at the AIDS Quilt."

"I'll think about it. Hey, by the way, why the hell's Rumpel even allowing it now? I mean it's a symbol, really, of America at its worst. And I know he wants to erase all that."

"I heard his sister begged him. Her husband died of AIDS in 1990. I read it in our printed underground, *No Stalin for Us*."

"I would like to read that one. I miss you Terri. And Leslie and June. And Mom."

"Maybe we can change all that soon. Merry Christmas, Soph. I love you."

"Love you too. Buon Natale."

MARCH 19, 2021
Birmingham Medical Center, Alabama

Sam Smith was the sixteenth patient to be admitted with bad diarrhea, high fever, and cough over the past few weeks. His wife, Reba, had been bugging him to go to the hospital for at least a week but he kept balking on account of the bad burn he had on his left hand. He did not want any doctor meddling in his business.

MARCH 1, 2021
West Side Women's Clinic, Birmingham, Alabama

They waited until the medical staff entered the clinic but acted before any patients arrived. Each of them lit two coffee cans filled with plant fertilizer providing the ammonium nitrate that would ignite with the fuel oil, and threw them in the rear door.

As Sam Smith and Calvin Cotton drove away, Sam struck a match for the cigarette he held in his mouth. A small flame emerged from his left hand. He must have spilled some of the coffee can liquids when he tilted them to light the rope fuse soaked in the dangerous mixture. He grabbed his handkerchief from the upper pocket of his bib overalls and killed the flame, but it left an awful mark on him.

When Reba asked him how he hurt his hand that evening, he said he must've got some of the fertilizer he had been sprinkling in their vegetable garden on his hand before he lit a cigarette.

She was not really listening to him, though, because the reporter on TV was interviewing the only doctor who survived the bombing at the abortion clinic early this morning.

"Whoever done blown up that place, Sam, did lots of hurt.

One doctor and two nurses is dead. Thanks God there wasn't any girls in there."

Sam smiled. He felt like he saved some babies today. White ones, that is.

March 20, 2021
Atlanta, Georgia

Burt Williams was thankful he was not sick on this warm Saturday evening as he said goodbye to his wife, Betty Ann, in Jackson, about one hour south of Atlanta.

"You be careful now, Burt, gett'n into the city."

"Sure will. Should be home in the morning, right in time for church, sweetheart."

He had told Betty Ann his charity for blind albino children was having a meeting in Atlanta. All the Georgia boys and even some Alabama ones usually met a few times a year, so Betty Ann did not think much of it.

But there was no meeting now because Sam was sick, and George from all the way down in Darien was still recovering from his hospitalization last month. All of them kept in touch through an online chat room they had named "Blinded by the White."

Burt took whatever opportunity he could, and he had not had any since last Halloween weekend, to stop in at that special bar in Atlanta. There he could be with "real men" who still believed in the cause of the antebellum South.

He pulled into the parking lot. The neon sign flashed: "JD's," and in smaller letters underneath it: "Southern Gentlemen Welcome."

To the right of the entrance another sign read: "Y'all be courteous now and keep your hoods lowered."

MARCH 17, 2021
Georgetown, Washington, D.C.

Ronnie Lynch was a junior at the university. It was Spring Break but he did not run off to the Bahamas, like many of his classmates did, because he was not interested in having that kind of a good time.

He was expected to go into law so he was majoring in political science. And he was expected to follow his father, Ronald Lynch, Sr., Vice President of the United States, into a political career.

Ronnie was supposed to hold his father's political and religious beliefs, and he did, for the most part. He was conservative, he went to church and believed what he heard there, especially about how homosexuals are sinners. He was proud his own father played such a big role in outlawing gay marriage again. But he only could discuss his feelings with the few other students at the university who felt the same way.

Even more so than his father, Ronnie liked to stay connected to the family's Southern roots that tangled deep down to a slave-owning family in Mobile, Alabama. Ronnie found "Blinded by the White" serendipitously, he felt, while searching the internet for a connection.

The chat room was secure. All guests had to enter a name to gain entrance. Ronnie made up anything he thought might get him in.

"Lynch man." Denied.

"Little Ronnie Reagan." Denied.

"Confederate Jack." He was in.

He loved the conversations. They talked about the really important matters, like how to make things in America better again. For starters, the white race cannot die, they said. No more abortions, they said. No more gays, they said. And definitely, no more immigrants.

Burt Williams, alias R. E. Lee, mentioned a bar in Atlanta named "JD's," just right off of 85 before Downtown. It was a place where American men could discuss these things in person.

Ronnie Lynch, alias Confederate Jack, thought he might have a bit of fun, after all, on this Spring Break. He would head down to Atlanta this coming Saturday night. The one Secret Service man assigned to him would have to follow in his car.

MARCH 20, 2021
JD's, Atlanta, Georgia

Burt Williams had been nursing a beer for the last hour when he spotted the college boy wearing a button-down shirt under a cashmere cardigan, blue jeans, and leather loafers.

"That boy has no business in here," the man sitting next to Burt said.

"Well now, he don't know no better."

"I'm R. E. Lee," Burt said when he reached Ronnie who was standing at the other end of the bar trying to order a drink. "You must be Confederate Jack."

"Hey, how'd you know?"

"Are you kidd'n me boy. No one else dresses like that in here."

"They do in Atlanta. I looked it up."

"We're in our own world in here, Jack. Let's have a drink."

Burt bought two bourbon and Cokes and led the boy to a quiet booth away from the bar.

They talked a long time about immigrants taking jobs like

the one Burt had as a shelfer in the local merchandise center down in Jackson.

"Some Central Americans filled our last two openings," Burt told him. "Their food stinks up the lunch room, I tell you that much, Jack."

Ronnie said he was afraid the same thing would happen to young men like him getting degrees, not that he had anything to worry about himself. Then they talked about the one solution for all of America's problems: producing more white people.

Ronnie finally was with someone who saw the world in the same way.

They were holding hands across the table now.

Burt said, "We can feel real proud to be white men and make our women with child and still have a little fun ourselves." He winked and swept his head in the direction of the curtain.

The bar closed at 3 A.M. Burt and Ronnie were the only ones left there when they walked out from behind the curtain. The bartender said good night and turned off most of the lights.

Outside in the soundless night of the parking lot Burt said, "Now look here, kid, if you're ever down this way again when we have one of our ceremonies for the sake of all of them children killed in them clinics, give me a call. We'll be sure to have a pig for Christmas again."

Burt handed him a JD's napkin with his cell number written on it.

Ronnie Lynch was not sure what he meant by the "ceremony" but it sure sounded interesting to him. He waved goodbye as Burt headed for 85 South. Ronnie thought it was real neat Burt's license plate read, "61-65 JD."

"The years of Davis' presidency," Ronnie said out loud and then pulled out onto 85 North. The black car was right behind him performing his job of protection.

MAY 17, 2021
Georgetown, Washington, D.C.

Ronnie Lynch knew his finals would be rough this semester but this was ridiculous, he thought. One week of diarrhea carried him to the last exam today in his WWII history class.

He was tired of answering questions about the Holocaust as his cough grew deeper and deeper and sweat dripped down into his eyes and onto the paper booklet. Other students were starting to throw him dirty looks.

When he handed in the dampened exam, his professor said, "You might want to visit a doctor, Mr. Lynch. We hope you did not share your microbial wealth with us today."

Ronnie called his mother. An ambulance arrived at his apartment within minutes. They took him to Crystal City. He was given plenty of IV fluids and oxygen for the two-hour ride that should have taken only 30 minutes.

MAY 18, 2021, NIGHT SHIFT
National Health Center, Crystal City, Virginia

Dr. Gerald Brugge should have been retired by now. He was 68 years old and actually did try it six years ago. He and his wife, Myra, an Art History professor, spent the first three months in Europe, starting in Prague and working their way back west to England.

Myra had lost 25 pounds in the last few weeks of their adventure. Gerald knew they did a lot of hiking in the Swiss Alps, but not that much. And he was concerned with the dull, gnawing pain in the left upper quadrant of her abdomen she only mentioned on occasion. He knew it was there most of the time.

He took her in for a diagnostic work up at the National Cancer Center that was still open then. The diagnosis: Stage IV Pancreatic Cancer.

Dr. Brugge knew there was nothing available to really help his wife. Immunotherapy had been practically curing other cancers but not this one. Myra died two months after her diagnosis.

Gerald was thankful she was at home with her pain controlled, and with their children who eased her passage out of this world.

Gerald tried travel on his own and spent his time oil painting, like he had wanted to do for years, but none of it sustained him. He returned to medicine four years ago.

The National Infectious Diseases Center had closed, but the one hospital left in Crystal City was thrilled to have him. Gerald did not miss the old days, anyway, watching patient after patient go to the grave no matter what he prescribed. But he did remember how proud he was to have overseen the first clinical trial on protease inhibitors that were so important in arresting the power of HIV back in the '90s

Gerald was content now to work nights. He never slept more than an hour at a time when he was home anyway. And he was happy to get interesting cases from time to time, such as that patient last summer who had just moved his family from Arizona to Fairfax, Va. The man had high fevers and quickly went into respiratory distress.

After interviewing his wife, Gerald discovered they recently took in a docile prairie dog as a pet. Gerald tested the man for *Yersinia pestis*, commonly known as bubonic plague and carried by prairie dog fleas out West. Seven days of IV Tetracycline cured the patient and seven days of the antibiotic in its oral form prevented the patients' wife and children from getting the bacterium.

And now the Vice President's own son admitted to the respiratory unit here with a nexus of symptoms that could just be coincidental or add up to some known syndrome or even a new one. Gerald felt a tinge of excitement and almost felt 30 years younger working on the diagnosis.

The admitting doctor on the day shift ran HIV tests first on Ronnie Lynch and all of them were negative. The diarrhea was still bad: ten times per day with the strong anti-diarrheals. No DTO was to be found here, but Lomotil helped.

The stool and sputum cultures were pending. Gerald knew it probably was not tuberculosis. Ronnie's cough did not produce the white pinkish-tinged froth, and the sound of it leaving his throat was not the high pitched lingering ring of TB that Gerald would never forget.

The antibody test for *Mycoplasma* did come back positive this night. So Gerald ordered Doxycycline IV, an old drug, yet the most effective one to treat this type of pneumonia. And now it looked like Ronnie Lynch's kidneys were starting to shut down. If the drugs Gerald ordered tonight did not make his kidneys work by the morning, dialysis would be necessary.

This all felt like a common viral source to Gerald. The only way, he knew all too well, to even begin to figure that out was to see if there were any other cases like Ronnie's out there. There was no weekly newsletter from the Central Disease Bureau where he could look now, ever since its circulation was banned. Any report of infectious diseases made America look bad, dirty, the president thought.

But Gerald still had contacts at the CDB. He waited until 8:01 A.M. for one of his oldest ones to arrive in his office, Dr. Jack Durante.

"Jack. It's Gerald. Gerald Brugge," he said when the phone

was answered.

"Gerry. Don't be so formal. How's retirement been treating you?"

"That's a story for another time. I've been back at the National Health for a few years now."

"They're lucky to have you, Gerry."

"The CDB is darn lucky to have you too. It's a shame though we don't have the weekly. It kept all of us connected."

"We miss putting it out, Gerry. But I don't mind talking to docs in the field about what's going on. It's usually manageable, but lately there's been a lot of activity."

"That's what I wanted to know about, Jack. I have a VIP, we'll leave it at that. He's a 21-year-old male with a one week history of severe diarrhea, high fever, cough, and now a diagnosis of *Mycoplasma* pneumonia. Have you had anything like this reported to you?"

"Interesting, Gerry. We've been tracking some cases locally, isolated to Georgia and Alabama until now."

"How many?"

"Yesterday, we just hit 101."

"What's the demographic, Jack?"

"All white men. All middle aged. All HIV-negative. All the symptoms you just gave me. Oh, but yesterday we had a report of kidney failure in Birmingham, Alabama, with the patient's second bout of *Mycoplasma* pneumonia."

"Well, as far as I know, Jack, this is my patient's first bout but he just developed renal failure yesterday, too. Any organisms coming back in the stool?"

"No."

"This sounds viral, Jack."

"A familiar feeling indeed, Gerry."

"Thanks a lot, old friend. I'll be in touch."

"I'll be right here. Just like last time."

MAY 18, 2021, 8 P.M.
National Health Center

Gerald Brugge was back on duty. The day doctor had been waiting for a call from Vice President Lynch that never came. When he did call, the unit secretary found Gerald discharging a patient in a room.

"Dr. Brugge here," he said when he picked up the phone.

"This is Vice President Lynch. How's my boy, doctor?"

"Stable but still in critical condition. We had to start dialysis today, for his kidneys."

"That sounds serious. What does he have, Dr. Brugge?"

"We're not sure yet. I mean we know he has pneumonia that's responding to antibiotics. His fever is just about gone. The diarrhea has slowed but it's still too much. And now the kidneys. I think it might be viral. It could be something new. It is not HIV...."

"Of course not. Ronnie's a good boy," the Vice President interrupted the doctor.

Gerald rolled his eyes and continued to explain. "Anyway, HIV tests are negative. There is no CMV, or mono, or hepatitis. Has Ronnie taken any new medications lately, that you know of?"

"No, doctor."

"Did he have any childhood cancers?"

"No, doctor. Have you seen anyone else with this ... illness?" the Vice President was hesitant.

"As a matter of fact, Mr. Vice President, there have been several cases reported to the CDB, Central Disease Bureau, over the past few months."

"What do they think?"

"It looks viral but we need to study more than your son to find the culprit," Dr. Brugge explained.

"I have permission already from the President to do whatever it takes to get my boy well again. What do you need?"

"To begin with, we should transfer any cases admitted elsewhere to the NHC here. We might be able to find some patterns, some other similarities."

"Do whatever it takes, Dr. Brugge. The government will take care of it."

"Thank you, sir."

"One more thing, doctor. Keep a tight lid on this. No press releases. No responses either if they start digging."

"Yes, sir," Gerald hung up the phone.

May 19, 2021, 8 A.M.
National Health Center

Gerald called Jack Durante again at the CDB and left him a message asking him to call his cell whenever a hospital notified the Bureau about any established or new patients with these symptoms.

May 24, 2021, 7 P.M.
National Health Center

Gerald arrived a little earlier tonight hoping he could catch the day nursing supervisor, Ashley Smith, before she went home. She was young but knew how to run a tight ship with the limited staff she oversaw at this hospital.

Ashley was still in her office coping with the budget. She needed more nurses but she needed the approval from on high for their salaries and for the bonuses she wanted to offer any potential candidates.

"Ashley Smith, Nursing Supervisor," she said when she picked up the phone.

"Ashley, it's Gerald. A great opportunity just fell into our laps."

"Let's hear it, doc."

"The V.P.'s kid is not the only person with this disease."

"That's great! I mean not about Ronnie Lynch and anyone else with it but if we have others to study.... It must feel like when AIDS started, Gerald, doesn't it?"

Ashley never really took care of any AIDS patients. She was born in 1990, but she had a keen interest in infectious diseases. She was honored to work with Gerald Brugge, one of the original AIDS doctors at the NHC.

"So, look, Ashley," Gerald said without acknowledging her last comment. "My colleague at the CDB tells me there are four patients like Ronnie just hospitalized."

"It's nice, Gerald, you still have your connections."

"We need to transfer them here, to the respiratory unit where Ronnie is. There are two in Birmingham, Alabama, and two in Savannah, Georgia."

"Why there?"

"That's what I'm hoping to find out."

"I can transfer some of my nurses from other units with low censuses right now. But I will need money for them, for their flexibility."

"The V.P. told me the sky's the limit. Offer them extra pay as well for the risk of exposure and for all the conversations they will be having with them to find the common thread."

"They will be safe, right, Gerald? I mean it seems like they will be. You and the nurses now have not gotten sick in caring for Ronnie Lynch."

"That's why we implemented universal precautions all those years ago, Ashley. Plus, I have asked all staff to wear gowns and masks with Ronnie until his *Mycoplasma* antibodies are negative. Just in case also, if there's something we haven't found yet."

"Perfect. They'll be on duty when the transfers come in. When will that be, Gerald?"

"Within the next 48 hours."

"Six nurses will be enough, right Gerald?"

"For now."

MAY 29, 2021, 6 P.M.
Dinkens International Airport, New York City

Sophia Maria Lorenzo's plane landed at 4 P.M. It only took her two hours to get through Customs.

"You're American, Ms. Lorenzo?" the Customs officer asked when she reached the glass enclosed booth.

"Yes. I was born in the Bronx. You can see my birthplace on my passport," she said as she handed him her booklet.

"How long have you been in Italy?"

"About three and a half years."

"Why do you live there?"

The truth would not do. Sophia had anticipated this question on the plane.

"I help young American girls living abroad keep their babies or get them adopted by couples in the States."

"What kind of babies?"

"White ones, of course."

"Welcome back to America, Ms. Lorenzo," the officer said as he stamped her passport.

PART 2

DUTY CALLS

May 26, 2021, 7:15 P.M.
National Health Center, Respiratory Unit

The Medevac helicopter touched down in Crystal City. Reba Smith was transported with her husband, Sam, who was very sick now. His pneumonia was not responding to the antibiotics that helped his first bout in March.

He was in complete kidney failure and had been receiving dialysis for a few days. Later this morning, he completed the four-hour procedure that filtered out the toxic waste products in his body before the helicopter battered the air in its slow ascent above Birmingham Medical Center.

May 27, 2021, 6:30 A.M.
National Health Center, Respiratory Unit

George Johnson from Savannah General, now with his second pneumonia and a skin rash not seen by any doctor before, should have been flown here but Dr. Robin Wake and the Savannah team thought he was stable enough for the eight hours of ground transport. He arrived shortly after Sam did. His flared nostrils and bluish nail beds indicated his lungs were not absorbing the oxygen he received through a face mask during the entire trip.

Bart Sawyer, who bought Sam Smith's other piglet shortly after last Halloween, had been admitted two days ago to Birmingham Medical Center with unstoppable diarrhea. His doctor there reported his case to the CDB because he could not isolate the source of it.

Bart arrived around midnight after an ambulance ride where he sat on a portable commode steadied between the ambulance stretcher and the metal wall the crew had lined with blankets to protect him from any bumps on the road.

Buddy Miller from Clayton, Georgia, about two hours north of Atlanta, was the last admission around 2 A.M. He was transported by ambulance from Atlanta Central Medical Center, the only patient with this new disease there to date. The combination of diarrhea and *Mycoplasma* pneumonia prompted his doctor to report his case to the CDB. Buddy was by far the healthiest of all the men now housed on this unit.

Dr. Gerald Brugge had two Infectious Disease fellows, doctors in training for this specialty, helping him with the History and Physicals and all of the orders that needed to be entered in the computer system for all four patients.

The three nurses on duty tonight had to collect the blood, stool, and sputum the doctors ordered for these men, in addition to performing and writing their own physical and psychosocial assessments; administering medications, IV fluids, oxygen, and breathing treatments; and changing their linens as needed with the help of two good nursing assistants.

Only now, near the end of their shifts, the nurses took a

quick break with cups of much-needed coffee. Charlene, almost 65-years-old and ready for retirement, found a low-key position on a geriatric unit at NHC a few years back and was not happy at all with this transfer assignment. She was not complaining too much, though, because of the hefty pay differential Ashley Smith offered her and the other nurses.

She was talking to Charlie, a 71-year-old Viet Nam veteran and nurse, not ever thinking about retirement, who had been working in the surgical ICU here that did not have any patients over the past month on account of the new private hospital, Special Surgeries Center, that had opened in nearby Fairfax, Va., about how sick George Johnson was.

"I sure hope the extra $50 an hour is worth it if I get Lord knows what from him," she said.

"Come now, Charlene. You know as well as I do it's darn difficult to get anything but some sweaty scrubs underneath all that protection we're using. Hell, we've been around a long time, and we never got any HIV or hepatitis, now did we, girl?" Charlie responded.

"That's right. I know. It's just these men are so sick. It's hard to know where to start caring for them and ourselves. Gloves go on for the rash. Mask for the coughing. Gowns for the splashing of Lord knows what," Charlene said.

"Well, that's just it. At least you two have an idea," Amy the third nurse said, "with decades of experience caring for patients this sick. I've only been on the orthopedic unit since I graduated three years ago and I've never seen anything like this."

Amy was only 25-years-old and had been overwhelmed with her assignment this shift. She admitted Buddy Miller, the easiest patient, and also cared for Ronnie Lynch who was stable on dialysis. But now his skin started showing the same purplish rash George Johnson had. She could not bring herself to touch it even with gloves on.

"But," Amy continued, "I'm just so thankful to you Charlene for taking care of Johnson, as sick as he is, and to you, Charlie, for taking care of Smith. I really would not even know where to begin with him."

"You listen up now, little missy," Charlie said with a leftover twang of Tennessee. "You come right on in with me to look Smith over from head to toe, after we finish this deserved cup of coffee, of course. I'll show you what to look for when something's not right with your patient, and if you need to inform Gerald, Dr. Brugge. And then I'll show you what needs to be in place for the oncoming shift. Last thing you ever want to do is not have your fluids in and out recorded, a fresh bag of IV fluids hanging, dry sheets, and a good turn of your patient one last time so he's not in the same position for too long bringing on a bed sore."

The day shift nurses started to prepare themselves mentally for a tough shift as they listened to report. Tina had the most experience, becoming a nurse on a Medical-Surgical unit with plenty of AIDS patients right before HAART was available in the mid-1990s. She took Sam Smith who was still breathing on his own, but not easily. She was ready for the worst since she had been a medical ICU nurse for years now.

Kristi was ten years younger than Tina and had a dialysis background. So Ronnie Lynch suited her just fine. And she took Buddy Miller whose pneumonia was beginning to respond to the antibiotics already.

Margarita had only been nursing for a few years but she was so eager to learn and care for really sick patients. George Johnson and Bart Sawyer surely would keep her challenged for the next 12 hours.

Dr. Gerald Brugge entered the break room as the two shifts

were finishing up report. Gerald wanted to ask the nurses if they could find some answers to a list of questions he compiled that might open some avenues of investigation for the under-lying pathogen he thought was circulating in the bloodstreams of all of these patients.

Gerald knew if anyone could get essential information from patients, it was the nurses. That was always how it was in the old days with AIDS when patients did not feel comfortable talking about who they were. He almost envied the relation-ships the nurses formed with all of them back then.

He began. "I asked George Johnson last night, when I admitted him, if he had done anything differently lately in his work or social life and he just shook his head no without even thinking about it.

"So it may take some time to find some answers to the following questions. But I know if anyone can do it, all of you can."

He wrote with a black erasable marker on the white board on the wall to the right of the coffee pot.

"Have you had any new sexual partners? If so, how many?"

"I can just see asking Johnson that one with his wife sitting there next to him in her Sunday best," Charlene interjected.

The other nurses laughed and Gerald smiled before he continued to write.

"Have you used any drugs recently? Have you used needles or straws to take them? Did you share?"

Gerald said he hoped the next question could identify the common source of infection.

"Have you traveled anywhere new, especially outside of the USA, in the past year? Where?"

Amy and Margarita copied down every word verbatim in their notebooks while the more experienced nurses said, "Got it."

May 29, 2021, 6:45 A.M.
National Health Center, Respiratory Unit, Staff Lounge

Gerald ordered a big breakfast tray from his favorite D.C. deli last evening for an early delivery this morning. Egg on brioche, bagels with cream cheese, pastries stuffed with fruits, orange juice, and dark roasted coffee welcomed the nurses in their breakroom.

Gerald was the doctor on duty last night so he knew how bad the shift was. Sam Smith went into respiratory failure and could not breathe on his own. He had a tube inserted down his throat that was connected to a ventilator machine. Gerald decided to keep Sam on this unit because of the isolation he required, plus he had the one-to-one nursing care he would have received in the ICU anyway. Supervisor Ashley Smith agreed with the doctor's decision.

Sam Smith had spiked a temperature to 104 degrees Fahrenheit last evening before his breathing got worse, and he had been losing weight fast, about 12 pounds in the last 48 hours. Gerald knew the fluid balance could be challenging in dialysis patients, but this was more than a typical weight fluctuation of 2–5 pounds daily.

When Gerald read Sam's chest x-ray last evening, it looked like he had PCP, *Pneumocystis carinii* pneumonia. "What the hell's going on? This guy does not have HIV and has not received any chemotherapy, but his immune system is under attack by something," he said to his ID fellow standing with him.

"Good morning," Gerald said as nurse after nurse hurried into the breakroom and grabbed something to eat from the enticing tray.

"How's it been going?" Gerald said after he gulped down some coffee.

He heard a lot of sighs and "Oh gods."

"These are sick patients. I know."

Charlie started talking about Sam Smith. "I thought it was strange, and it's hard to believe I even ended up noticing it with everything else going on with him, but he has a darn bad burn on his left hand that needs some care itself. I've been using Silvadene cream."

"It looks like it's been there for a while," Gerald said. He told Charlie he also noticed it before Sam went on the ventilator and asked the patient about it. Sam told him he hurt himself with plant fertilizer. Gerald then said he got too busy trying to control Sam's breathing problems to ask him any more questions about the burn.

Charlie added, "Yeah, that's what he told me too. I pressed him for more information and he said his hand caught on fire when he lit a cigarette after sprinkling some fertilizer on his vegetable garden back home.

"Then I asked Mrs. Smith when the burn happened and she said back in March. The only reason she even remembered that was Sam told her about it when she was watching the news about the abortion clinic bombing in Birmingham then."

"I remember that," Gerald said, and a few of the nurses said they did too.

Tina, Sam's day shift nurse, had entered the breakroom a few minutes ago and heard what Charlie said before he had to go back out and relieve the nursing supervisor, Ashley. She was standing outside of Sam's room ready to alert one of her nurses if the ventilator alarmed.

"Well maybe Sam Smith did burn his hand on the plant fertilizer in his garden or just maybe he had something to do with that clinic bombing."

"Why do you say that, Tina?" Gerald asked.

"Because I looked up what those bombs are made of and that fertilizer is one of the ingredients. And every time Mrs. Smith cries about how sick Sam is she always says he's such a good man, always trying to help those albino children.

"When I asked her what the organization was that he helps, she said, 'I don't know what theys named for sure but I know my Sam wants to save as many as he can. That's why he's always cursing them clinics where them white babies always die.'

"Then I asked her if she meant abortion clinics and she nodded yes. Then I said not only white women have abortions you know. And she said, 'Theys do in Alabama.'"

Charlene added, "She may be right about that one, Tina. I know even my people, up in Connecticut, tend not to terminate."

"I didn't realize that," Tina responded.

"I'll tell you what I didn't realize. That's how prejudiced these people are from the South, at least those deep in it, like Johnson."

"What did he do to you, Charlene?" Margarita was a little afraid to ask her.

"It's what he doesn't do. He does not look at me. He does not talk to me, and I know damn well he talks because I hear him telling his wife how to fix his pillows and anything else he needs."

"I'm glad it's not just me," Margarita said. "I asked his wife if I did anything to offend him because he will not look at me or talk to me either. You know what she said? She said, 'He just prefers his own kind.'"

"I hope that doesn't mean what I think it does," Tina said.

"I think it does, Tina. And I couldn't help myself. I told

Mrs. Johnson that I am his kind. I am a human being and an American just like him."

"What did she say then?" Charlene asked smiling.

"Not a thing. But I don't know if that's worse or what Mr. Sawyer did last evening before I went off duty when I was helping him back to bed from his commode for the eighth or ninth time.

"I felt so sorry for him with his diarrhea not slowing down in the least until ..."

"Until what, sweetie? Tell us, Margarita," Charlene said. "It's OK."

"He pinched me right here," she pointed to her buttocks. "He said, 'All you Puerto Ricans are ruining this great country. But there's nothing wrong with tasting a little brown sugar now and again.'

"I grabbed his hand and I told him, 'I am Mexican, Mr. Sawyer. My parents came to America before I was born. I was born here just like you, and it seems like you need me taking care of you right now more than I need you.'"

"That a girl, sweetie!" Charlene said. "You have much more patience, and courage, than me. After the assistant, Cheryl, and I changed Sawyer's bed when he could not make it to the commode last night, he said to me, 'Much obliged *Nurse*.'

"Then under his breath I swore I heard him say the *n* word."

"I couldn't believe it, but Cheryl heard it too. I can't remember the last time I was called that. I haven't been back in his room since, and that happened around 1 A.M."

As Gerald listened to the nurses' experiences throughout the same shift he worked, he was still amazed how they always managed to see the real person behind the patient lying in the bed.

"So, to recap. Sam Smith might be an abortion clinic

bomber fueled by white nationalism. And George Johnson and Bart Sawyer are awful racists.

"Racism is a pretty big thread uniting more than these patients, unfortunately, in our country right now. But this is not giving us any other clues, yet.

"Any other stories we should hear?" he looked at all of the nurses.

Kristi started talking about Ronnie Lynch. She said he was sad. She said no friends ever came in the early evening when visitors usually do, plus he never gets any phone calls except from his mother.

Kristi then mentioned Ronnie's father came to see him the other day, "a three-ring circus with all that security. Well, Tina and Margarita were there." They shook their heads and rolled their eyes.

"Anyway, I feel bad for the young gentleman with no friends and powerful parents who are essentially absent. And now the dreadful purplish lesions on his torso that don't seem to be fading. And it's almost summertime now."

Then she asked Gerald, "Hey, Dr. Brugge what did the biopsy results show, the one you took on that back lesion of his?"

"No cancer at least," he said.

Kristi said she took some time and sat next to Ronnie near the end of yesterday's shift. "It's uncomfortable though, in all that protective garb, and I didn't want to stay in there too long in case I catch something."

"That's highly unlikely, Kristi," Gerald said.

Kristi did not reveal the next part to the room because she knew her beliefs were different than most nurses she knew.

She had talked with Ronnie awhile about how she was happy, like he was, that his father helped to ban gay marriage again. "What was this country thinking, letting men marry men and women marry women? Next thing you know someone can marry a sheep or a cow," she told him.

As Ronnie started to open up to her about a girl he was interested in in his political science class this past semester, Kristi asked him if he asked her out. She would be a fool not to accept, with him being so handsome and now 21-years-old, Kristi thought.

Kristi did share the next part of the conversation with the breakroom.

"Ronnie Lynch told me he hadn't done anything with anyone no how. I told him it was nice talking with him and he smiled. Then in the antechamber to his room, after I degarbed and scrubbed my hands and face so vigorously I thought I was going to bleed, I noticed the Secret Service man, always stationed outside his room, staring at me.

"When I came back out to the hallway, he handed me a napkin, a cocktail napkin, and said, "I don't know what Lynch has told you but this might help. It was his only adventure over Spring Break."

Kristi took the napkin out of her scrub jacket pocket and passed it around to all of the nurses. It finally made it to Gerald who read it out loud:

"JD's
Southern Gentlemen Welcome
Rt. 85
Atlanta, Ga. 30324"

JUNE 1, 2021, 6:30 P.M.
National Health Center, Ashley Smith's Office

The nursing supervisor had hired some agency nurses to help cover shifts on the respiratory unit during the times when the transfer nurses were off.

These nurses earned double the high hourly wage of the transfer nurses but still only signed two-week contracts when they heard about the isolation requirements for this unit, instead of the month-long ones Ashley usually arranged when she got desperate enough to utilize this expensive staffing option.

And these nurses were ready to leave already.

"What are you saying, Julie?" Ashley asked the nurse who came to see her before her shift ended. "You've only worked two days. Do you think you might want to delay any decision until you've fulfilled your contract at least?"

"Ms. Smith, I can't take all that coughing and crapping. It's like those AIDS patients back in the '80s."

"Was it really that bad back then?" Ashley asked.

"Oh no. It was much worse than this, Ms. Smith. But I never wanted to work with them, no one did really, but they kept showing up on the Med-Surg unit I worked on in D.C. I didn't have a choice then, but I sure do now."

"I see," Ashley said.

"Of course, I'll finish my two weeks but I'll be moving on after that."

Two other agency nurses stopped in to see Ashley before they gave report to the night shift. They said there was too much exposure to "Lord knows what" and no amount of money in the world was worth all that.

JUNE 3, 2021, 6:30 A.M.
National Health Center, Nursing Supervisor's Office

Ashley had been coming in early and leaving late with all the staffing issues on the respiratory unit. And they were not letting up.

Kristi was coming on duty and knocked on her cracked-open door.

"Hey, Kristi. Come in. How's it going? I hear you've been doing a great job with Ronnie Lynch."

"Well, thanks, Ashley. I feel like he's starting to trust me. He's so afraid and no one is around much at all. His mother comes in once in a while after her important lunches, but still no friends. And that older man from Georgia, Buddy Miller, he's all alone too."

Buddy had talked to Kristi for almost an hour yesterday morning about how his wife left him for a younger man last year. He told Kristi, "Can you believe after almost 25 years of marriage she up and left me for one of them Mexicans."

Kristi responded, "I know what you mean, Mr. Miller. My boyfriend did the same thing to me. It's no wonder our country is the way it is."

Kristi did not repeat this part of the conversation for Ashley, but she did tell her supervisor that Buddy's pneumonia was resolved.

And then she said, "It's weird how we cannot isolate any bacteria or virus in his stool. All those cultures are negative. I mean we just don't know what the diarrhea is coming from. It's kind of scary."

"You are wearing gloves, right, Kristi?" Ashley asked.

She shook her head yes.

"And a gown when you come in contact with any fluid?" Ashley asked.

"I'm still wearing a mask, Ashley, even though Dr. Brugge said we don't have to ever since he took the patient off of respiratory isolation."

"So why are you still wearing it?"

"I'm so afraid, Ashley. When I go home at night, I shower for at least an hour and even that's not enough."

Ashley was starting to get concerned as she listened to this nurse.

"I need to go back to my old unit. The worst I can get there is hepatitis. I'm vaccinated for hep B, and C is curable now with medicine, as you know. But this. We don't know what any of this is."

"Can you hold on a few more weeks, maybe a little longer until Dr. Brugge is closer to identifying a pathogen in these men?"

"I can't, Ashley. Oh God. I don't know that I can do another shift. I'm just going to have to quit."

"No please, Kristi. I'll send you back to dialysis tomorrow. Just go up to the unit today and give me this last one," Ashley said and hugged her.

Tina was waiting on the other side of the door when Kristi came out.

"Please don't say it, Tina."

"I'm sorry, Ashley. It's horrible taking care of these men, and I've only had one of them who can't even talk on the ventilator."

"So, what's going on, Tina? You are an experienced intensive care unit nurse," Ashley said.

"I know. It's not the pneumonias Sam Smith has, or the diarrhea, or the purple lesions covering his body now. They look a little like Kaposi's Sarcoma, but Dr. Brugge said they're not. I don't care anyway. I've taken care of my fair share of KS in the past."

"So, what is it, Tina?"

"I can't stand who these people are."

Tina said it's even worse than she thought. She had

suspected Sam Smith might be an abortion clinic bomber but now she was pretty sure he was a member of the Ku Klux Klan.

"His wife told me more yesterday. I wish she hadn't."

Ashley's eyes looked eager to hear but afraid to know.

"Mrs. Smith started talking about that charity of his, for the albinos again. I asked her how Sam helps these children exactly. She said first of all Sam and the other men try to feel how the children do. I asked her how they do that.

"She said, 'Theys wear white hoods so they can feel their blindness.'

"I asked her where they wear these hoods.

"She said, 'When all the men are together theys drive to events for them children.'

"I asked her if they drive with their hoods on.

"She said, 'Deed I see Sam drive off with it on. Yes ma'am.'

"I then asked her how they can experience the blindness of those poor albino children when they must be able to see through those hoods when they drive. Otherwise they would crash their cars.

"She laughed a little then and said, 'I sure don't know for sure, nurse, but I know theys like to feel like those poor children do.'

"Then I asked her if she would like to get a cup of coffee in the visitor's lounge down the hallway, and I asked one of those agency nurses to keep a close eye on Sam.

"Have you ever considered Sam could be a member of the KKK?

"She said, 'I don't know about all that, nurse. Them clansmen sure do bad things to them people and I know Sam don't care for them at all. I don't think he's ever lynched any of them though, not that I know about anyway.'"

Tina then told Ashley it felt like the Civil War and the Emancipation Proclamation never happened every time she was in Sam's room, and she was in there twelve hours a day with the exception of a quick break here and there.

"Ashley, my daughter's biracial. My ex-husband is Black. All of this with Smith got me thinking about how hard it was dating him in the 1980s. People were awful then. I just thought the country was trying to get up to speed with the Civil Rights Movement two decades before that.

"But in Sam Smith's world none of that ever happened. He is one horrible man, a real racist. And Mrs. Smith is equally horrible in her complicity."

Tina also mentioned all of the ugly comments Margarita endured from George Jonson and Bart Sawyer.

"Geeze, Tina, why didn't she switch patients with Kristi?" Ashley asked.

"Are you kidding me, Ashley? Ronnie Lynch and Buddy Miller are just as bad, but Kristi doesn't mind."

Ashley decided not to ask why. "Can I expect Margarita next, Tina?"

"No way, Ashley. She's a good one. She manages to place all of her patients' horrible beliefs in a box, that's how she described it to me, so she can focus on taking care of their sick bodies.

"I admire her but I can't stand another minute of this kind of hatred. Please, Ashley, transfer me back to the ICU," she said and stood up to go on duty upstairs on the respiratory unit.

JUNE 3, 2021, 6:30 P.M.
National Health Center, Nursing Supervisor's Office

Charlene was coming on duty again tonight but got off the elevator on the second floor of the wing where the respiratory unit was to look for Ashley Smith's office. Charlene had made her work home the geriatric unit years ago so that she never needed to find this office.

"Ms. Smith. Good Evening," Charlene said after she gave a little knock on the half-opened door and Ashley said, "Come in."

"Oh, Good Evening to you, Charlene. At least I hope it's a good one."

"I'm not so sure about that, Miss Ashley."

"How has it been going for you? I know it's been hard taking care of these men."

"Indeed, it has been, Miss Ashley. I even switched assignments with Amy last night hoping that would make a difference."

"But it hasn't, has it, Charlene?"

Charlene had thought Ronnie Lynch, who she knew went to school in Georgetown and was exposed to a more diverse student body, would be more open-minded than George Johnson from all the way down in Darien, Georgia.

And last evening Charlene thought Ronnie particularly would be on his best behavior after his father's visit. She thought he still would be wearing the public persona as the son of the second most powerful person in America.

Charlene felt bad for this young man as she hung his antibiotic after giving him another diuretic to help shed the water accumulation in his legs. She knew after reviewing the most recent chest x-ray and lab results after his dialysis today that Ronnie's pneumonia was improving but not his kidneys.

"How are you, Mr. Lynch. I'm Charlene, your nurse for this evening right on through to the morning. You tell me what you need and I'll make sure you get it," Charlene said to him as she did her work with him.

"Where's Amy? Where's my *real* nurse?"

"Amy is taking care of some other patients tonight, Mr.

Lynch, but I can assure you I've been a nurse for more than 40 years now."

"Is that so? I didn't think you people were allowed to go to college back then."

"I can assure you, Mr. Lynch, I did and I have been practicing nursing ever since then."

"I know you can't possibly be as intelligent as Amy though. We have proof of that," he said.

Charlene did not hold back in repeating this conversation for Ashley now.

"How on earth are you supposed to care for someone who says that to you at the beginning of your long 12-hour shift, Charlene?" Ashley said.

"Well, I did. It was certainly no easier or harder than it was caring for Buddy Miller. He's from north of Atlanta so I thought it was going better than it did with Bart Sawyer from way down in Alabama, until I helped him into the bathroom."

"What happened then?" Ashley asked like she was listening to someone describe a movie scene.

"Well, I know how sore Mr. Miller was from all that diarrhea and I wanted to help him feel better with a good sitz bath."

"What's that?"

"Miss Ashley, how long have you been a nurse?"

"Less than ten years."

"How long did you take care of patients?"

"Only two."

"Lord have mercy. For people with real sore rear ends we place a basin under the toilet seat and hang a bag of lukewarm water that runs through a tube into the basin. The water swirls around while the patient just sits there and it helps to soothe all that rawness," Charlene explained.

"I missed a lot, wanting to get into administration right away, Charlene. But I don't mean to interrupt."

"So I was walking behind him to the bathroom in case he fell and I could catch him. But he couldn't hold it in until we got there. Most of it hit the floor but some of it got on my shoes.

"Next thing he says is, 'I've never had no brown person see my private parts before. I'm sure you people like it though just like them damn Mexicans do, 'specially the one doing God knows what with my wife now. She left me for one. Can you believe that?'

"Yes, I can, Mr. Miller. Now let's get you cleaned up and on that toilet for a little comfort."

"You mean you still helped him, Charlene?"

"Of course, I did, Miss Ashley, but that's it for me. I need to go back to my unit or somewhere else after tonight's shift. I can't take no more abuse from these men. It feels like the Civil War hadn't even happened yet when you're with these men."

"That's pretty much what Tina said too, Charlene," Ashley had to comment.

"And I'm not going to lie to you, Miss Ashley. I'm tired of all of the exposure to some bug we don't even know about yet. I didn't want to do it back in the day with AIDS and, Lord help me, I sure don't want to do it now. I've almost reached my retirement.

"You have a good evening, Miss Ashley," Charlene said and went upstairs for what she knew was going to be her last shift on the respiratory unit."

Ashley was starting to pack up her briefcase when Amy, the second youngest nurse she transferred here from the NHC's orthopedic unit, knocked on her open door with tears in her eyes.

"What's wrong, Amy?"

"It's 18:55, I only have five minutes to make it up on the unit. But I can't take it anymore."

"Tell me, please, Amy. Sit down."

"Last night Charlene and I switched assignments hoping it would be better for her with Lynch and Miller instead of Johnson and Sawyer."

"But it wasn't. She told me."

"It wasn't any better for me either, Ashley, not this assignment or my old one. I mean, honestly, I'm a white girl from South Carolina and I'm offended by the language these men use."

"Do I need to hear the particulars, Amy?"

"No. I mean it's plum terrible the way they talk. And they think because I'm white and Southern that I look at everyone else who is different from me like a wild animal that needs to be caged.

"That George Johnson's the worst of them, I tell you. And the sicker he gets, and he's pretty dang ill with that purplish stuff on his skin growing wider and deeper and his pneumonia not going anywhere, the meaner he gets.

"And now he keeps talking about pigs and how the next one they get will really help all of them save those white babies."

"What does he mean by that, Amy?"

"I don't know but it's not good and I don't want any part of it anymore. I want to have babies of my own one day and I don't care if my husband is brown or Black or blue just so he's a good man who I can love and he loves me back.

"But I ain't going to get there taking care of these men with their horrible illnesses we don't know nothing about yet and their horrible hearts and minds."

It was now 7:15 P.M. Ashley asked Amy if she could make it through this shift at least.

"I think I can, Ashley."

"Can you give me until next week to transfer you back to

your unit or somewhere else if orthopedics doesn't get more admissions over the weekend?"

"I'll go anywhere, Ashley. Anything's better than this," Amy said and left the office.

"What the hell am I going to do now?" Ashley said out loud and paged Dr. Gerald Brugge.

JUNE 3, 2021, 9:00 P.M.
National Health Center, Respiratory Unit, Doctor's Lounge

"It's not a good sign you're still here, Ashley," Dr. Brugge said as she closed the door behind her. "I'm sorry I couldn't leave the floor. I need to be available if Sam Smith crashes. He's not doing very well."

"How much worse can he get, Gerald? He's on a ventilator," Ashley said.

"Well his oxygen levels are down. His *PCP* pneumonia is not responding to Pentamidine. I'm switching him to good old Bactrim. It used to work the other way around with our AIDS patients back then."

"That doesn't sound good, Gerald. And now I have more bad news," Ashley said while she plopped down in a big, cushiony armchair many medical residents dozed off in when they took call.

She told him about the agency nurses first.

"So we have them for how long?" Gerald asked.

"Another week. They signed two-week contracts."

Then she told him about the NHC transfer nurses.

"How many want to leave?" he asked.

"Four of them. Two on nights and two on days."

Gerald asked if it was the racism they had to deal with or the isolation precautions.

"Both," Ashley said. "Except for Tina. It's just the racism. She thinks Sam Smith could be KKK. Mrs. Smith told her that her husband wears a white hood for his charity work for the albino children."

"Unreal," Gerald said. "But I wish I knew what that had to do with his illness and these other men."

"You should know, Amy mentioned something really strange in caring for George Johnson. He said something about how the next pig will help to save the white babies."

"What the hell does that mean? Pigs and babies. Any ideas yet about cities, or states, or even countries where these men have been, Ashley?"

"Well, you remember Kristi gave us that napkin from a bar in Atlanta."

"But that was only where young Ronnie Lynch has been. Anyway, Ashley, who's left?"

"Charlie on nights and Margarita on days."

"I'm not surprised Charlie is staying. He's seen a lot and much worse than any of this stuff back in Nam."

"You mean Viet Nam. That horrible war, Gerald?"

"Yeah. He fought during the worst of it, in '68--69. I was not old enough for that tour of duty. Thank God," Gerald said.

"I did not know that about Charlie. My grandfather fought during that time, too. He died from cancer last year. His doctors said it was all that Agent Orange he was exposed to then."

"It's caused a lot of stuff we're still dealing with today. I am surprised, Ashley, that Margarita is staying. She's brave for her age. And I know the patients have been downright abusive to her."

"They sure have been," Ashley said. "Now who else am I going to get to take care of these men?"

"Can't you hire more agency nurses or transfer some more nurses to this unit?"

"I can't transfer anyone right now. All of the other units are starting to reach full census. And I've been calling every agency I know ever since the first agency nurses started to visit me in my office. News travels fast, though, in nurse circles. I'm hoping to find anyone to sign a contract who hasn't heard about all of the particulars of caring for these patients."

Gerald had been looking at the ceiling as Ashley told him about her staffing woes.

"It's crazy what I'm thinking, Ashley."

"I'll take anything, Brugge."

"What we need are nurses who don't mind caring for patients who may be contagious, even though they've proven not to be so far, and who don't mind wearing masks, gowns, and gloves. And nurses who don't even mind removing all of it too when it's safe, of course. That always helps the patients be more like themselves. Then we might get more information to figure out all of this.

"And what we really need are nurses who can put aside their own beliefs, their own politics, and just care for these very sick patients."

"Tina said that's what Margarita does. She places all of the patients' beliefs in a box and puts the box up on a shelf for the shift. That's kind of what you mean. Someone's beliefs need to be stowed away when they're so different. It doesn't seem to matter if it's your own or the patient's. But Margarita--- and I'm guessing Charlie does the same thing--- are the only two who can do that, Gerald. I don't know that I could," Ashley said.

"I know I can't, not for 12 hours straight in their rooms," Gerald said.

Gerald knew exactly who they needed. The problem was many of them were dead, or too old, or not practicing, or too battle-worn to come on duty once again.

"Ashley, did you know the AIDS Quilt will be on display this Saturday on the National Mall?"

"I sure did, Gerald. I can't wait to see it."

"You might feel differently when you do. It's darn over-whelming looking at that sea of the dead with every name being read out loud non-stop."

"What does the Quilt have to do with the nurses I need, Brugge?"

"It's a long shot, Ashley. I know that. But if we could get some of them to come and help us to find the clues to this virus or whatever pathogen is infecting our patients."

"But how do you know any of them will be there?"

"My guess is since the president says this is the last time he will allow it to be displayed, and it is the 40th anniversary of the first AIDS cases, many of them will be there. Well, I say many but there were never many, not outside of San Francisco and New York. Even in those cities there were handfuls of designated AIDS units where nurses volunteered to work."

"I did not know that, Gerald. I thought every hospital had an AIDS unit."

"They should have. We at least did here at NHC, when we had the Infectious Diseases Hospital. But all those nurses left long ago, many before the ARV revolution and the rest after it. It was rough back then."

"How will we meet them, Gerald? I mean there are going to be millions of people there. And any kind of public notice, as you know, has been banned unless it's approved by the government."

"I'm thinking we should use small cards, like place cards at a dinner party, inviting them to meet with us. We can place them under, or between, some of the panels in the Quilt."

"That's good, Brugge. Maybe I'll get neutral colored cards

and use a light blue ink so we draw just enough attention, but not too much."

"That sounds good, Ashley."

"So, I guess we can't ask for them to meet us right there at the Quilt because that might be considered organizing. So where should we ask them to meet us, Gerald?"

Ashley continued to answer herself. "*The Smithsonian*, maybe. I've always loved it there. It houses all the best we value as humans. That would be appropriate, wouldn't it?"

"That's a good idea, Ashley, but I think *The Holocaust Museum* will speak to those nurses the most."

"That's intense, Gerald. What do you want the cards to say?"

"What do you want them to say, Ashley?"

"How about:

AIDS Nurses: Your Expertise is Required
Meet and Greet with NHC
The Holocaust Museum, Shoe Exhibit
Saturday, June 5, 2021 @ 7 P.M.

"I'll get the exact address of the museum for the cards later."

"That sounds great. Why the shoes?" Gerald asked.

"There are always lots of people there, and we won't stand out. And as you said, Gerald, there probably won't be too many of them anyway. I hope there's enough, though."

"You'll be there with me, I hope," Gerald said.

"I wouldn't miss it for the world. It's one thing working with an original AIDS doctor, it's quite another to meet, and if I'm real lucky, work with some original AIDS nurses.

"I watched that film a few years ago about the very first ones in San Francisco. It was amazing what they did," Ashley said.

"We'll need to get to the Mall before dawn on Saturday, Ashley. I have a special pass to enter and leave when I want to. They gave one to all of the old timers at NHC. And the memo sent to us said the Quilt panels will be arranged geographically with West Coast names on one end and East Coast on the other. It also suggested we could spend some time at the microphones reading names.

"As far as I know, there's no reason we can't touch the panels. So, we can split up, Ashley, and place some cards near the edges of each coast of names. It'll just look like we're kneeling down to pay tribute. I'll be doing some of that anyway."

"It's a date, Gerald."

JUNE 4, 2021, 8 P.M.
Train from New York City to Washington, D.C.

Sophia and Terri had boarded the 6:00 P.M. Mercury, the high-speed train system built on the East Coast under President Bahama. Congress had approved the funds for the tracks and electric cars to extend out West, but Rumpel derailed that money to off-shore oil drilling and resurrecting the deep-lying embers of the coal mines.

Sophia returned to America now because she feared, even if Rumpel was not president one day, the AIDS Quilt, this moveable Holocaust memorial, as she saw it, could be destroyed for good.

Sitting next to her sleeping sister, she was thinking about how much she enjoyed her time with her mother over the past week. Mrs. Lorenzo was almost 80 years old, but that did not stop her from gobbling up any piece of authentic news, meaning any news not approved by the President of the United

States. She could not wait to read the underground papers Terri delivered to her every Saturday morning.

Sophia thought her mother probably shared the recent healthcare developments she had read about with her yesterday afternoon because of where she and Terri were headed tonight.

Walking along Arthur Avenue in the Bronx to Alfonso's, still serving the best panettone, and the best cannoli they were in search of for tonight's dessert, her mother began.

"Sophia, did you know the president issued an executive order allowing doctors and nurses to refuse to take care of people if they do not agree with their beliefs, or choices, or who they are."

"The president tried that in the '80s, remember Ma, but the Supreme Court upheld the equality care law. What the hell?" Sophia said.

"Suppose your sister gets in a car accident and is really hurt. Suppose her doctor objects to her being gay? Who's going to help her?" Mrs. Lorenzo said as they walked into Alfonso's.

"Ma, you're turning into an activist."

"Keep it down now, Sophia. It's hard to know who you can trust, she whispered. "Morning, Vinnie. I need a dozen cannoli. How's your wife?" Mrs. Lorenzo asked the owner who was picking out the nicest looking stuffed pastry shells for her.

"Thanks a lot, Mrs. L. She's feeling alright this week. That chemo stuff didn't bring her down too much this time," he said.

"I'm glad, Vinnie. See you soon," Mrs. Lorenzo said as they walked away.

"What kind of cancer, Ma?"

"Ovarian."

"Oh."

Sophia was listening to the lull of the train skating along the tracks feeling proud of her mother. She even put Diego in his place when he came to dinner last night, alone. Giada had asked him for a separation after this past Christmas holiday. She told him she needed more from him emotionally.

Mrs. Lorenzo, Sophia, Diego, and Sophia's niece, June, were enjoying Mrs. Lorenzo's signature lasagna and Sophia's pasteles that she stuffed with pork because she knew Diego liked the classic form, when Mrs. Lorenzo raised her glass of wine to toast June's parents.

"Here's to Terri and Leslie's sixth wedding anniversary. I hope they're having a nice dinner."

"There's no real anniversaries for the queers, Ma," Diego said.

"You stop that nastiness, Diego, especially in front of June. And you remember she's my daughter, your sister. Their marriage has turned out to be so much better than yours anyway. Giada has tried but you haven't grown with her, worked on it. You could learn a thing or two, heh, from your sister."

Boy, she really gave it to him, Sophia thought and laughed a little waking up Terri.

"Hey Ter. I'm going to get a cup of coffee," Sophia said standing in the aisle now.

"Try and choke it down, sis. You're not in Florence now."

"You want one too?"

"Not a chance. Even I have standards."

Sophia was looking out the window in the refreshment car sipping her coffee with lots of cream she added trying to get it to taste better.

Something about the rusty highlights in the sleepy sky reminded Sophia of nights long ago when she and Sura would sit in the breakroom after report was over with their first cups of coffee from a new pot, the envy of all the other hospital units for its sharp smell and taste, and smoke another cigarette and look at the big bridge through the window before going out to the floor to begin the long night of giving medications for infections no one had ever heard of before AIDS, adjusting oxygen tubes and masks, administering breathing treatments, and then turning them together, changing their sheets, holding their hands, and listening to how their lovers or friends or parents had not been around to visit them lately or at all.

The now of 2021 and the then of 1989 folded into one moment. Sura was standing there in front of her.

"Do you remember that one night before we started when David was shouting in that high-pitched voice of his and we had to leave our cigarettes and our coffees earlier than usual?"

"I do, Sophia."

"Do you remember what he needed?"

"A screwdriver," Sura said laughing. "That poor man thought he was at a bar instead of sitting on the floor next to his bed with his legs crossed."

Sophia finished the story. "'How long does a gal have to wait to get a drink around here?' That's what he said when we helped him back to bed."

"I remember it well, Sophia."

Sophia stood up. She was afraid to hug her. But once she did, she did not want to let go.

"My God, Sura. How are you?"

"I'm just fine, sweetheart. How are you?"

"I've been living in Florence, in our apartment, for more than three years now."

"I know. I keep up with you through your sister. We are in the museum all the time. I love the Egyptian rooms. I always bump into Terri there."

"She's here with me, Sura. How's Harold?"

"He died in 2012, in his sleep, thank goodness."

"I am so sorry, Sura. He was a wonderful man."

"I'm here with Liz. We married in 2016."

Sophia smiled. "You're one lucky gal, Sura. You got two good ones in one lifetime."

"Yes, I am."

"I assume we're headed in the same direction, Sura."

"I never thought I could do it, Sophia, especially after the last time I saw you."

"I barely remember that, Sura. I did not stop drinking for months. I went to the liquor store around the corner on York Avenue after the coldness stung every inch of Ricky's dead body lying so still in our bed.

"You visited me after the service. It was all such a fog."

"I did. You were not in a good way."

"But I interrupted you, just like I always have managed to do, Sura. You were saying."

"I never thought I could see the Quilt." Sura explained that anytime she saw Sophia, and it was not that often since 1995, it always brought back so much. So when the Quilt was on display in its entirety in 2011 for the 30th anniversary, Sura felt like if she went to see it she would not be able to pull herself back to the present, to life.

"I didn't think I could ever do it either, Sura. But when Terri told me at Christmas time that it would not be on display again, I felt like I needed to see it, to pay homage to all of them, what they went through, what we went through with them."

"Do you think we'll come back from it all, Sophia?"

"I hope so. I'm glad we'll do it together."

"Yes. Where are you staying, Sophia?"

"The Lincoln Hotel, not far from the Mall."

"We're booked there too."

"Let's get a taxi together at the station," Sophia said.

June 5, 2021, 6:10 A.M.
The National Mall, The AIDS Quilt

Ashley was waving and running when she saw Gerald standing at the foot of the Monument facing the reflecting pool.

"I'm sorry I'm a little late. I was up until 2 and overslept," Ashley said through quick breaths.

"I should've offered to help you. My age and ego preclude me from recognizing when I'm an awful chauvinist. My apologies, Ashley. How many did you make?"

"Around 60."

"Thank you so much, Ambitious Ashley. I can see you as a director some day at NHC."

"We'll see about that, Brugge. Right now, I'm worried about finding some nurses to staff my unit who will stay long enough until we find the culprit of this disease," Ashley said while turning to the other side of the Monument.

She was looking at the green mall layered with what looked like one huge, seamless blanket stretching into the rising soft yellow sun. "My God, Gerald. All of them are dead?"

"Yes."

"All those families without their children, their spouses, their partners, their siblings. How did you do it, Gerald?"

"I don't know. We had to. Someone had to."

"Let's get busy, Brugge," she handed him half of the cards.

June 4, 2021, 9:45 P.M.
The Lincoln Hotel, Washington, D.C.

Terri was so glad Sura and Sophia bumped into each other on the train. She knew Sophia would be OK at least with one of her own by her side.

The four of them were having a light dinner with Caesar salads, a little wine, and some sparkling water. Terri and Liz talked while Sophia and Sura got caught up on the last decade or so of their lives.

"This must be hard for Sura," Teri said.

"It is. It will be. All of this brings back her childhood too. It's hard for me to understand completely. I'm an American Jew, raised in New Hampshire," Liz said.

"I know Sura is from Germany."

"Yes, Düsseldorf."

Sura Weber's mother was German Jewish and her father was just German. Her parents married in 1930 and Sura was born three years later, the year Hilter became Chancellor.

"The Nazis made these 'mixed marriages,' as they liked to call them, illegal by 1935," Liz explained.

"I remember reading about it, in college," Terri replied.

"She remembers Kristallnacht," Liz said.

"My God. She was young," Terri said.

"Five. That's why when she talks about it, it's all fragmented."

Sura's parents thought they would be safe in the synagogue in the town square when everyone got word that the Nazis were coming in November 1938 to arrest Jews married to non-Jews, Jews who still did business, and even Jews seen dining out in public or going to the theatre.

Liz said, "She remembers hiding under the floor boards in the synagogue all day and all night. That's why to this day she can't stand to be in complete darkness."

"Sophia used to tell me Sura bought nightlights for all of their patients' rooms. She never told Sophia why she did that. Now I understand," Terri said.

Liz continued, "The Nazis broke anything they could find in homes, shops, and the synagogues. Sura says sometimes in the middle of the night when she can't sleep, she still hears that awful noise. The sound of big fish tanks shattering over and over again."

Sura also told Liz that before that night she used to hear her parents talking about some camp at Dachau. Her parents said it was a labor camp, but they always ended any mention of it with "Well, that's what the government says anyway."

"It's very telling now, Terri, that Sura responds to anything she reads or sees about the processing of undocumented immigrants at our borders with, 'Well, that's what the government says anyway."

"I can see why," Terri said and ordered another glass of wine, and so did Liz in this musty Victorian lounge, one of the oldest in the District.

Liz told Terri about Sura's grandparents, her mother's parents, the Lichtensteins. They always served Sura small sips of the ale her grandfather brewed by trade, and chewy, crusty pretzels baked by her grandmother.

"All those memories stopped, though, after Kristallnacht."

Liz then mentioned the map Sura's mother kept in the kitchen above the table on the wall. She placed a red pin on any area where someone she knew had seen her parents. The last pin was placed on Bergkirchen, about five miles from Dachau. A Düsseldorf jeweler Sura's mother knew met a brewer in Munich while conducting his own illegal business. This brewer knew Sura's grandfather and had spotted Mr. Lichtenstein on an open train headed for the labor camp.

"Sura memorized that map, I tell you, Terri. She knew the position of all of the pins where her grandparents were after she never saw them again. She went to all of those towns about a decade ago, and then found their names, Harvey and Sura Lichtenstein, on the rolls at Dachau."

"My God," Terri replied.

A few minutes after 11 P.M., Sura touched Liz's arm and said she was exhausted.

June 5, 2021, 10 A.M.
The AIDS Quilt, The National Mall

The four ladies had breakfast later than they intended, but the croissants, fresh strawberries, and dark roasted coffee were just enough to carry them over to the Mall. It was the first cup of coffee Sophia had without cream since she arrived back in the States.

Sura and Sophia were looking across the length of the Quilt now. They reached for each other's hands to begin the long walk to the East Coast panels as each name creeping through the microphone struggled to secure its place in the air.

"Are you OK, Sura? I mean do you want some help to get there?" Sophia said.

"I may be old, Sophia, but I was on this side of the fence also when we worked together back then. I still remember some nights when I ran circles around you."

"You sure did, Sura. I just wanted to make sure."

"I know. Thank you. I do not need a wheelchair to carry me. You'll do just fine. And I'm right here for you, too."

Sophia smiled as a tear fell down her cheek. She used to not be able to cry at all, about anything for years, when she worked on the AIDS Unit and for a long time after that.

The first time she did was the night Ricky died and then she couldn't stop. The wine helped her but it turned against her in the end like it always did.

After a month, she returned to her counseling job at the Lower East Side Women's Center, but it took another two months to return to sobriety. That happened when she bumped into one of her patients at a wine bar in midtown.

When she moved to Florence, Sophia would cry a little whenever she started to think about those days, about what she and Sura were facing right now together. And she did find a good therapist who helped her begin to scrape the surface of these old wounds.

They knew they reached their side of the Quilt when the panels displayed pictures of the World Trade Center and the Empire State Building, Independence Hall and the Liberty Bell, and the Capitol stitched around, above, and below the names of the dead.

And then they really knew they were home when they saw Cal, Calvin Moore, still a rail thin nurse they worked with on the AIDS Unit at The Upper East Side Medical Center for about four years, a fellow soldier indeed.

Cal stood up. He looked more comfortable, more settled now, as the woman he always wanted to be. Cal started talking to them like it had been 30 days since she had seen them last instead of 30 years.

"Look at our Eduardo, little Eddie, right here, beautiful ladies," she said as she pointed at the panel. "I managed to serve him the most unsavory cup of juice when I was running around trying to get everyone's AZT into them on time that night. Lord, those four hours came around fast.

"Tom told me, our beloved aide, Tom. He told me he had just filled up everyone's pitchers with fresh water and their favorite juices right before my med rounds."

"Oh, I remember, Cal. You thought it was apple juice over ice. And when you gave it to Eddie with his pills he said it tasted like piss," Sophia chimed in.

"That's because it was, girl!" Cal snapped her fingers up

high. "That poor thing had dumped his juice in the garbage can and used his pitcher to piss in. Who would've ever thought.

"Now you two come here. Girlfriend needs some hugs and kisses."

The three of them held each other a long time. And then Cal said, "I've been here under an hour and I swear we know every other poor soul in this section. Was it really that many?"

"Should we split up to see all of them? I don't want to miss anyone," Sophia said.

"Let's stick together you two," Sura said and Cal nodded her head. Her sunglasses were hiding reddened eyes.

They tiptoed around the panels. Sophia spotted Mrs. Miranda Lopez's quilt and bent down to touch it. She thought of the daughter sewing pictures of her mother's favorite foods from back home on the quilt while holding it in her lap during her long visits. And then she saw one of the cards left by Ashley and Gerald.

"Hey you two, what do you think this is?" Sophia held it up and read it:

AIDS Nurses: Your Expertise is Required
Meet and Greet with NHC
The Holocaust Museum, Shoe Exhibit
1945 East Wiesel Drive, SW, Washington, D.C. 20003
Saturday, June 5, 2021 @ 7 P.M.

"That's interesting where they want us to meet them," Sura said. "I've been meaning to get there. I'd like to see something, anything, from Düsseldorf where I was born. I just never thought I would be facing two Holocausts in one day."

"You really see it that way, Sura?" Cal asked.

"I do. The discrimination, the neglect, the denial of people being exterminated."

Then Sophia said, "You know when I think about the night Mrs. Lopez came in, Sura, what you're saying really rings true."

Sophia started talking about the tiny, elderly woman from Guatemala who had been admitted with *Cryptococcal* colitis when she was on duty. Sophia and the aide, Tom, made sure her bed was well-padded and she had a diaper on because she could not hold in all of the liquid that insisted on coming out.

The worst part was how confused Mrs. Lopez was, which only Sophia understood because of the language they shared. Sophia figured the virus was probably in her brain already. Sophia had asked the patient's daughter how long her mother was sick.

"Too long, Dios Mios.' Then the daughter explained over the past year her mother had lost 50 pounds. That was after the hip replacement surgery back home in Guatemala.

"There were complications after the surgery. 'Blood loss,' her daughter said, 'and she needed a blood transfusion. That's where the SIDA came from.'

"But Mrs. Lopez's family, her daughter told me, called her 'puta' and 'mala' when she got sick. That means whore and bad, bad person, if you want the exact meanings."

Sophia went on. "I don't expect you two to remember, but I was the only nurse on that night she was admitted. Her daughter asked me and Tom if we could put a little jacket restraint on her because of her confusion.

"She said Mrs. Lopez was usually up all night talking to her father who had been dead for a few years now. She said she could not stay the night, but sure wanted to, because she had to watch her grandson when her own daughter went to work at the bodega all night up in the Bronx, not far from where I'm from.

"I hope Tom and me are forgiven for what happened next.

We had her tucked away in bed for the night. It was 2 A.M. and we needed a break, the first one since we came on duty at 6:00 P.M. Just one cup of coffee and a cig, and a few bites to eat of Chinese food we ordered from across the park hours ago."

"Where was the second nurse for you that night, Sophia?" Sura asked.

"You remember some of those nights. We didn't have anyone else. No one to transfer. Well, hell, that never worked out anyway. No one ever wanted to work with our patients. The supervisor said we were just fine with me and the aide for only six patients," Sophia explained.

"Yeah, honey. Like that was OK. Those six were like taking care of 12 patients anywhere else. They were sick, sick, sick," Cal commented.

Sophia continued. "And then we heard it, boy. 'Ayuda! Ayuda!' Help, Help, she did not stop and it was so loud it woke up even our patients who slept around the clock. We ran to her room. Mrs. Lopez's body was still in the bed restrained in that jacket, but her head was almost on the floor.

"And her right leg, the one without the hip replacement, was caught in her bedside rail. It was turned completely around. We didn't know it until we pulled her body back in the bed and she screamed even louder. We could see then that her toes on that leg were pointed towards her back side."

Sophia said next she ran to the nurse's station to page the medical resident on call while Tom waited in the room with Mrs. Lopez. She explained what happened to the doctor and asked for him to come immediately. She also asked him to call surgery. But after 30 minutes there was no visit from the medical resident.

Sophia then paged the surgical resident. When he called her back, he said, "'What unit are you on?'

"The AIDS Unit on the third floor of the medical tower."

"'No emergencies there,' he said. 'We'll make our rounds later.'

"I'm so glad I at least got a morphine order from him. I gave her as much as I could to dull her pain. It was awful.

"At 0640, the surgeon finally graced us with his presence. He said, 'Hey, she's in pretty bad shape. Why didn't you page me again?'

"I told him. 'I did, doctor, every 30 minutes, to be exact, and the hospital operator has a record of all of my attempts.'"

"He said, 'Well, she's going to die anyway.'

"So, true, doctor, aren't we all, but nobody should suffer like that in the process, should they?" I told him.

"That was real good, girl," Cal interrupted. "I'm starting to remember all this now. You then helped him to manipulate her leg back into place after you insisted she had more morphine."

"That's right, Cal. And Mrs. Lopez sure was sore after that but not in pain. As I recall, she lived another month. I don't remember her suffering anymore."

"She did not, Sophia. I was on duty the night she died. It was peaceful. Her daughter was there and that adorable great grandson of Mrs. Lopez's just sitting at the foot of her bed rubbing her leg all night until she left this world," Sura said

Sophia held up the NHC invitation card again. "So, what on earth could they need us for?"

"I can guarantee y'all it ain't perdy," Cal said in her deep, Mississippi accent that Sura and Sophia knew all too well only surfaced when Cal got really nervous.

JUNE 5, 2021, 5 P.M.
Flanagan's Pub, Washington, D.C.

Sophia and Sura found Terri and Liz before they left the Quilt exhibit and headed to a pub near *The Holocaust Museum* for a bite to eat with Cal and her husband, Teddy. Teddy always knew the right place for the right occasion here in the District where he grew up.

Flanagan's on East Wiesel Drive had Shepard's pie and Beans on Toast for the Irish-minded or American style burgers and fries. Teddy could never resist a pint or two of the Guinness that tasted just like it did in Dublin.

Away from the bar, the two sisters and the two couples sat down at a big, round wooden table, the record of this pub's many visitors from around the world who had carved their names and homes on its surface.

It turned out that Sophia, Sura, and Cal were not the only ones with invitations to an event tonight. Terri and Liz showed everyone the index-sized flyers they found embedded in the West Coast and Mid-West sections of the Quilt. They would be attending the GC (Gay Coalition) meeting at *The Black History Museum* tonight at 7:30 P.M.

Terri commented, "I figured, and hoped really, the GC would have something going on during the Quilt Exhibit, especially since it's the last time anyone will be able to see it. It's been damn hard to meet anywhere back home in New York. It always seems like some mole manages to bust up our meetings, even though they're only advertised in our print newsletters that are not so easy to find."

"Why don't you post them in *No Stalin For Us*?" Sophia asked. "I've been reading the ones you give to Mom."

"Well, as you can see, Sophia, that's a more general underground for everyone and anyone who opposes Rumpel. Our newsletter is more focused. *The GC National* has been trying to organize meetings so we can get our people in place to try and stop the government from sending gays to the conversion centers, too."

"You're kidding, right? I mean you wrote me about them for the transgender, which I thought was horrific," Sophia said.

"I wish I was kidding. Rumpel is getting ready to sign another order to round up all the gays who have gotten married legally. That's how he'll start to identify us. Officials will search the marriage license databases."

"This is all much worse than I ever could have imagined," Sophia said.

"I just hope *The Black History Museum* isn't a trap for us," Terri said and Liz agreed.

"Oh, it's not," Teddy spoke up now. "I know Sherri who organized it. She told the scheduling secretary at the museum that the meeting was for gay people who came to Jesus, to the light, and had renounced who they were. The flyer at the museum says 'JC meeting tonight'."

"That's good," Liz said. "Will you be there, Teddy?"

"I wish I could be, but I organized an RLA meeting at *The Bible Museum*," Teddy said.

"How on earth did you manage that one?" Terri said while laughing.

"What's RLA?" Sophia asked.

"Right to Live with AIDS," Terri replied.

"I'm so out of the loop now," Sophia sighed.

Teddy thought the safest place to meet would be *The Bible Museum*. No one watching this weekend would ever think of seditious activities occurring there.

"I told the meeting scheduler that our group needed Jesus badly for ourselves and all of them poor babies not making it into this world. I told her we're Right to Life Alcoholics, recovering, of course."

"Damn, that's good, Teddy," Terri said.

"What does Right to Live with AIDS do now, Teddy?" Sophia asked. "I know back in the day, when we hardly had any drugs, all the activist groups fought hard."

Teddy explained after Rumpel got elected he kept his promise to bring down the cost of health insurance for all Americans by cutting coverage completely on all antiretroviral drugs to treat HIV.

RLA connects people with HIV/AIDS to the smaller pharmaceutical companies, such as Activitas, that manufacture ARVs, illegally, for a fraction of the cost of when these drugs were covered by insurance.

"The problem now, Sophia, is the damn government discovered Activitas' manufacturing facility and shut them down," Teddy said.

"So, no more ARVs? I guess, only for those who can afford them. That sounds familiar," Sophia said.

"Yup, it's not good. If we don't do something fast it's going to look like 1985 all over again. But there are other companies, like Sansvir, who are willing to make them for us. We just have to get the compounds to them. That's why we need the meeting tonight, to figure out all the logistics," Teddy concluded.

"I can't believe it's gotten so bad," Sophia said.

"Yes, you can, Soph. That's why you left, remember, when all of this began," Terri said.

"But it's so much worse now," Sophia said.

"What made you leave, sugar?" Cal asked.

"I had been working as an addictions counselor at a women's clinic for years and I had a girl who wanted to have an abortion right around the 12, 13-week mark. I could not find a doctor to perform it. I asked for qualified doctors I could refer her to in local newspapers and in medical blogs for women," Sophia explained.

"When was that girl?" Cal said.

"The summer of 2017."

"That's when things just started to get bad," Cal said.

"I know. I got a court sentence to attend speech therapy classes for my written requests to doctors to perform a procedure made legal by our Supreme Court decades ago."

"It barely is now," Cal said and continued. "It took a little longer, not much, for that kind of shutting us up in San Francisco. But they sure have now. The Castro used to have the sounds of protest all day and night."

"That's what I mean, Cal, in terms of how bad it is now. It's so quiet here in D.C. Silent really."

"Yeah, girl and you know what that means. Death, death, death," Cal said. "That's why we marched back then, isn't it?"

"That's why we took care of them," Sura added.

"Sophia, did you go to Italy with that handsome hubby of yours, the smart lawyer, 'deed a fellow Southerner? I remember when the two of you bought the place," Cal thought she could make the conversation lighter.

"I did go, but Ricky could not. He died in 2008."

"How absolutely terrible! I am so sorry. I had no idea. You are way too young to be a widow," Cal said as she reached for Sophia's hand.

"He had liver cancer."

"How unfair is that. A recovering alcoholic, and a faithful one, as I recall."

"Well, his hepatitis C did not care about all of that," Sophia revealed for the first time to people other than her family.

"I always take it for granted that we have the drugs now. Knocks that virus right out of your body for good. I see it all the time at the ID clinic, outpatient, of course, at Bay City General back home. I keep my hands in it," Cal said.

"I admire you, Cal. I don't know if I could do even that now," Sophia said.

"You sure about that, Sophia? You're one hell of a nurse," Cal said.

"She's one hell of a counselor too," Terri interrupted.

"I don't doubt that for a minute," Cal said.

"Did I hear there's a nurse amidst this fine-looking crowd?" a man with a chiseled face starting to give way to the softness of age asked in an Irish brogue.

"There are a few of us here, sweetie," Cal replied.

"I myself haven't tended to too many patients in a few fortnights, really years, to be sure, but when I did I toiled away at The Village Community Center in New York City."

"When was that?" Sophia asked.

"In the last century. The '80s and '90s. How about the likes of you?"

Sophia leaned into Sura and Cal and said, "We worked at The Upper East Side Medical Center during the same time."

"I'm starting to feel like all of us might have a bit more in common than the comfort of a good pint of Guinness in this fine pub," he said and raised his glass. Teddy did the same in return.

"Forgive me rudeness. I'm Jack, Jack Doherty."

Sophia and Sura introduced themselves and then Cal did. "Cal Moore here, but you can call me Cali, sweetie."

"Take it easy, Cal," Teddy whispered in her ear.

Sophia started to speak for all of them. "We were AIDS nurses then, Jack. Sura and I worked on nights together for eight years."

"I continued on another two after she left me," Sura said.

"And I worked four of those years, but on the day shift," Cal said.

"I was at Community for about 10 years, nights. I almost cracked completely, to be sure. I should've left before I did."

"I bet, Jack," Sophia responded. "You were on the first one in the city then. 1984, right?"

Terri said in Sophia's ear, "You mean first AIDS unit?" Sophia nodded her head yes.

"To be sure. I don't know what was worse, trying to comfort that young lot of them dropping like flies left and right, or fighting the hospital administration every day and night to get them to allow their lovers and friends to be at their sides."

"I thought about working down in the village on your AIDS unit but it was a Catholic hospital. No offense, Jack, but I had enough of it all growing up. The church dictating who's sinful when the priest themselves... I better stop," Sophia said.

"No offense taken. I'm in complete agreement. But I've always said it's better to dine with the devil you know than the one you don't."

"I like that sweetie," Cal said.

At 6:45 P.M., Jack gulped down the rest of his second pint of Guinness, in their presence anyway, and said, "I'm guessing we're all headed to the same meeting."

"We sure are, sweetie," Cal said and slipped her arm around Jack's as all of them left the table. And then she said, "You lead the way."

Cal turned back around to Teddy and threw him a kiss and a look that said, "I'll be good."

JUNE 5, 2021, 6:45 P.M.
The Holocaust Museum, Shoe Exhibit, Washington, D.C.

Ashley Smith stood there alone trying to process the mound in front of her. A docent walked, back and forth, the length of the room.

"Excuse me, sir. I came here when the exhibit opened last year. I thought it was the first time the shoes were here. But now I'm reading they were here in the early part of this century, and then went back to Poland. Why did they come back here again?" Ashley asked him.

"The museum thought it seemed most appropriate to have them on display now. It's been so hard to sort out what's true and not true these days."

"I see what you mean. The shoes are the physical proof that so many people, so many Jews, were murdered back then in the camps."

The docent nodded his head.

"I mean what other explanation is there for all of them? It's like the AIDS Quilt out on the Mall."

"Go on, Ashley," Gerald Brugge had been listening to her and the docent when he arrived.

"Oh, Hi, Gerald." The docent left the room after shaking Gerald's hand. "I mean every panel in that quilt is like every pair of shoes behind that glass. They are the record of human beings who died because of their differences from those in power. How horrible is that!"

"I'm impressed with your insight, Ashley."

"I do read books, Brugge, not just texts and Twitter feeds, you know."

"I did not mean to offend you, Ashley. It's just that your generation doesn't seem to know much about AIDS in the beginning, before all the drugs came along.

"Granted my experience with people your age is limited. The ones in training now in Infectious Diseases dismiss that time as the plague years out of the annals of medieval medicine.

"Even my own grandson, Brandon, almost 30 now, reads an awful lot. He's working on a PhD, on the history of epidemics in the U.S.A. But when he spoke to me recently about AIDS pre-HAART he acted like a time traveler to a bygone era."

"Well, Gerald, in some ways it is like that for us. We were just born as the AIDS drug revolution was underway. We did not learn too much about those days in high school. I never really did even in nursing school. Why focus on the past?"

"Not so much focus, but keep the bad years in mind right alongside all the good ones so we don't forget, and so we know what to do if it happens again," Gerald responded.

"Well, that's not going to happen, Brugge. We do have the drugs now," Ashley said.

"True. But you know the president took away coverage for all antiretrovirals treating HIV/AIDS."

"Yes, but people can still get the drugs on the market."

"What happens when they can't?" Gerald said.

Ashley now looked at him like she had looked at the shoes when she first arrived here tonight.

JUNE 5, 2021, 7:05 P.M.
The Holocaust Museum, Shoe Exhibit

Ashley saw an older group of people approaching them. She recognized the white older man with thick ginger hair and the Black grey-haired woman from that movie she saw about the first AIDS nurses in San Francisco.

"Oh my gosh, Gerald, I think they're here," she whispered

in his ear. Not that anyone could have heard Ashley since the music of Beethoven was piping through the room.

"What a coincidence, Gerald," Ashley continued to speak in a normal voice, "that the music began right when they arrived."

"Coincidence, maybe. Hopefully, it will ensure no one can hear us talking," Gerald said.

"But how did…. It did look like you knew the docent," Ashley said.

"Just an old family friend," Gerald said.

JUNE 5, 2021, 7:00 P.M.
The Holocaust Museum, Elevator to the Second Floor

They were all together. Cal was the branch connecting east to west. She had worked with Fred Johnson, the red-headed nurse Ashley recognized when they entered the room, for decades now in the outpatient ID clinic at Bay City General Hospital in San Francisco.

LATE 1995
Biloxi, Mississippi

After Cal left the AIDS Unit at The Upper East Side Medical Center, and he really felt like he had to then after turning HIV positive, he started pulling his life together. That meant no more leather bars, no more nights with men whose names he never knew, no more dressing up *like* a woman. Cal was going to *be* that woman.

The gender reassignment surgery was successful, which meant Cal was happy with her body, finally. Cal had it done in

Thailand by the American doctor there who had performed hundreds of them before and had no problem operating on anyone who carried the virus.

When Cal returned to the States, after months of recovery in Thailand, she went home to Mississippi first, now that her mother was dying from breast cancer.

Mrs. Moore was so happy to have her very own Cali back home. That's what she always called Cal as if she had been willing Cal's true self into being since he was little. Mrs. Moore always knew. Cali never played with other boys. There were no Western movies, no cowboy and Indian fights. Instead, she always found Cali with his sister, Lulu and her friends, donning boa scarves pretending to be movie stars.

Cal knew caring for her mother week after week that she was California-bound. Every time Cal visited San Francisco when living in New York he felt like he was leaving home flying back east. She would make San Francisco her forever home, and it could be now with all of the drug combinations flying out of clinical trials to treat HIV.

After her mother died, Cal ended up staying in Biloxi much longer than she intended, though. The week before she was supposed to leave for her new job in San Francisco, she had a few drinks with Lulu that turned into months of recovery and a permanent disability from the damage inflicted by the crowbar the men used to beat her outside of that bar. Cal had bumped into some old high school classmates who could not let "a dark freak run wild in the world," as they put it.

Lulu took Cal into her home until Cal could walk again, especially since their father, bitter from his wife's death but even more so from his thwarted dreams of being something, anything other than who he was in the deep South, could not refrain from using the word "disgraceful" every time Cal was in his presence.

When Cal left Lulu and the South for good, the job at Bay City General was still available. Cal's injuries only allowed her to take the position in the clinic part-time, but Fred was so pleased to have her.

Fred and Cal grew to be good friends outside of work. Fred and his husband, Li Yong, and Cal and her husband, Ted Young, were all neighbors in the Castro and tried to one up each other every Sunday night by taking turns preparing gourmet meals.

JUNE 5, 2021, 7:05 P.M.
The Holocaust Museum, Shoe Exhibit

Fred was holding Linda Washington's arm, the other nurse Ashley recognized from the film, as they approached the shoes. Linda had mentored Fred when he graduated from nursing school in 1984 and started working on the first AIDS Unit ever at Bay City General. Everyone called Linda the "AIDS avatar."

She had retired years ago but remained close to Fred. Cal knew Linda from their Sunday night dinner parties that she attended once a month, but she felt like she really did not know Linda at all, like there was a bolted door there she opened for only one or two guests at a time.

Back in the elevator, Cal had introduced Fred first to Sura and Sophia.

"I've heard so much about you two. Cal's rocks during those years," Fred said.

"You mean he never called us Scylla and Charybdis?" Sura asked.

"Maybe once, or a few dozen times," Fred laughed and hugged them both.

"I was never sure which one I was meant to be," Sophia said.

"It never mattered, darl'n. The two of you were strong, strong, strong together. For the patients, for me, for everyone really. Just don't try and cross the two of you," Cal said and snapped her fingers above her head.

Sophia and Sura laughed.

"Oh, and Fred, this is Jack. We just met him but he worked down in the Village on our first unit in New York City," Cal said. Jack shook his hand saying how nice it was to meet him.

"Well, NYC nurses this is Linda Washington, our very first," Cal said.

"What a pleasure to finally meet you, Linda. I'm Sophia."

"Thank you," Sura said and shook her hand.

"It's bloody good to meet the Eve of us all," Jack said.

Linda hugged each of them when they got off of the elevator before Fred took her arm, and said, "It's good to know there are still some of us out there in this world."

JUNE 5, 2021, 7:06 P.M
The Holocaust Museum, Shoe Exhibit

"Good Evening, nurses. I hope that's who all of you are," Ashley said as the six of them reached the shoe exhibit.

Sophia nodded her head yes and said, "NHC, right?"

Ashley smiled and nodded. "It's such an honor to meet all of you. I'm Ashley Smith. This here is Dr. Gerald Brugge."

"You ran the first protease inhibitor trial in '92 or '93, Saquinavir, I believe," Linda said. "We were one of your sites at Bay City General."

"A pleasure to meet you," Gerald said.

All of the nurses introduced themselves to Ashley and Gerald as three more people approached.

"More nurses, Gerald? We could be so lucky," Ashley spoke into his ear.

Linda hugged the still handsome, graying Italian-looking man, and Jack hugged the woman with bright red hair starting to ashen who seemed hesitant to return his gesture.

The very tall man in this new group was the first to speak, "I'm Thomas Bechtel. Good evening. I presume this is the NHC meet and greet."

"It sure is, Thomas. Thank you so much for coming," Ashley said.

"Hi, I'm Dan Napolina," the man who hugged Linda said.

"I'm Bridgette Delaney," the woman who Jack knew said.

"Hello nurses. I'm Ashley Smith, nursing supervisor for the medical division at the National Health Center in Crystal City, Va. This is Dr. Gerald...." Ashley stopped when she noticed Gerald was no longer in the room.

Sura had been standing away from everyone else staring at the shoes.

"Are you alright, Sura?" Sophia asked when she found her. "It's terrible seeing this. All of them gone. Thank goodness you and your family got out when you did, when you could."

"Not all of us did, Sophia. Liz knows what I mean."

"Tell me, Sura," Sophia said.

"My parents brought me to New York City after Kristall-nacht. You knew that. But my grandparents we never saw again before we left. They were last seen on a train headed to Dachau."

"Do you remember them?" Sophia asked.

"I do. They always made me feel warm inside. Soft pretzels baked by Oma and sips of tasty ale made by Opa. He was a brewer."

Gerald was back in the room now with the docent. "Mr. Lichtenstein here has found a room for us. This way please."

Gerald said to Ashley walking behind the docent," I am impressed so many of them came. Your cards were a great success."

Ashley smiled.

"Did he say Lichtenstein?" Sura asked Sophia walking behind Gerald and Ashley.

"It sounded that way," Sophia said.

"The surname of my grandparents," Sura said.

"You must speak to him, Sura," Sophia said. "Maybe he's related."

JUNE 5, 2021, 7:20 P.M.
The Holocaust Museum, Staff Meeting Room

"I love your connections, Brugge," Ashley whispered in his ear when they entered the room.

"Nothing special," he said.

"Maybe that's the way you see it, but this morning I had an exclusive preview of the AIDS Quilt and now this."

"Well, this many of us could not have stood around those shoes for more than a few minutes without raising suspicion. Honestly, Ashley, I thought maybe a handful of them would show up."

"It's really good, Gerald. Do you want to begin?"

"No, you should, Ashley."

"Hi again, everyone. In case you did not hear me out there, I'm Ashley Smith, nursing supervisor for medicine at NHC and this is Dr. Gerald Brugge, Infectious Diseases at NHC." Gerald raised his hand hello. "We're so thankful all of you came."

"What do you want to do with us, Miss Ashley?" Cal asked. "As you can see, we're all pretty ripened, for nurses."

"Some of us are practically fermented," Sura said.

"But like a fine pint of Guinness," Jack added.

"You said it, honey," Cal leaned into him laughing.

Ashley smiled. She was a little nervous. "But that's exactly why we need you. We have what looks like a new disease."

"What have you been seeing?" Fred asked.

"Patients with *Mycoplasma* pneumonia and lots of diarrhea. Oh, and renal failure and skin lesions they tell me look a lot like Kaposi's Sarcoma but are not."

"A multisystem disease. Interesting," Sophia said. "Like HIV."

"It's not though. They've all tested negative," Ashley said.

"How many are there?" Linda asked.

"We have five at NHC, all on our respiratory unit," Ashley said.

"What's their demographic?" Jack asked.

"All white men, middle aged, mainly," Ashley said.

"Well, that's changed a little," Gerald added while Sophia jumped in. "Is there any drug use or unprotected sexual activities involved?"

"We're not sure about that yet," Gerald responded. "But we do know from the CDB that there are more than one hundred cases out there all sharing this cluster of symptoms Ashley just mentioned. They are all from Alabama and Georgia. All are white and male except for the female we just admitted today. And we have the first death."

Ashley's eyes widened. "What happened?"

"Ashley knew what I knew yesterday. We had five male patients with us. All white, four middle aged and one younger," Gerald explained.

"How young?" Sura asked.

"Twenty-one," Gerald said.

"So, what happened, Gerald?" Ashley asked again.

Gerald addressed all of the nurses at the table and explained that one of his ID fellows called him a few hours ago with an update on Sam Smith whose PCP pneumonia was not responding to Pentamidine or Bactrim.

"Wow," Sophia said. "This must be some bug."

"He died around noon," Gerald said and mentioned that his wife who had been by his side the whole time he was at NHC started having breathing problems right before he died.

"My fellow thought the patient's wife was just anxious, but the nurse kept saying she was not getting enough oxygen," Gerald said.

"That must have been Margarita," Ashley interrupted.

Gerald nodded and continued to tell them that Mrs. Smith was admitted with what looked like *Mycoplasma* pneumonia and pretty bad diarrhea causing her dehydration and fainting episode right after her husband died.

"I need to get to the hospital soon," Gerald said.

"Oh, that poor woman," Ashley said. "Her husband dies and now she's sick too."

"So, Dr. Brugge, it is Brugge, right?" Sophia asked

Gerald nodded and said, "Please call me Gerald, everyone, please."

"So, Gerald," Sophia continued. "Do you think this woman contracted the *Mycoplasma* through her close contact with her husband in his room or is it the sign of an underlying virus she's carrying?"

"Great question, Sophia. If she was going to get the pneumonia from her husband via droplets in the air when he coughed that seems like it would have happened during his first bout of pneumonia back in March."

"He was hospitalized then?" Sophia asked.

"That's what his records tell us. Then he was readmitted to Birmingham Medical Center in mid-May with pneumonia again and renal failure," Gerald explained.

"It could be sexually transmitted," Sophia said.

"Indeed, my friend Jack Durante at the CDB and I thought it sounded viral since the patients are so concentrated geographically and share the same cluster of symptoms. And now with the wife of one our patients coming down with it, too," Gerald said.

"So, Gerald and Miss Ashley, this is all really, really interesting, even mysterious. A real storm brewing again in the world of infectious diseases. And a southern one this time. Whooee! But what are we supposed to do?" Cal asked.

"I guess we should start by asking how many of you are willing to help us find some answers, really *the* answer," Gerald said.

"But why do you need us for that?" Linda asked. "Surely you must have plenty of nurses, young ones, to help with this new disease."

"Well, that's just it, Linda," Ashley began. "We don't. Well, we did, but we don't now. Really there are not a lot of nurses out there with your experience, your ability to care for a population no one else wants to touch or talk to even."

"Hell, what's so bad about them? You've told us the diseases y'all have been treating. They don't sound too bad to me compared to what we cared for back then," Cal said

"My nurses, well most of them anyway, don't want the risk of infection," Ashley said.

"We know a bit about that," Jack said.

"And also, it's what these patients are. Who these men are," Ashley said.

"What is that?" Sura asked.

"What are they rapists and child molesters, then?" Jack chimed in again.

"You might almost wish they were," Ashley said.

"So far, we think all of them are white nationalists," Gerald said.

"Like neo-Nazis, KKK?" Sura asked.

"One of the nurses who cared for the man who just died thought so. She also thought he was an abortion clinic bomber," Ashley said.

"Back then we took care of minorities, Blacks, browns, gays, transgender, drug abusers. We cared for the persecuted, not the persecutors," Fred said.

All of them shook their heads in agreement.

"What makes you think we would *want* to take care of these people?" Sophia said.

"Not *want* to, necessarily. But *can*. Most cannot. How many nurses have we lost on our respiratory unit?" Gerald said.

"Four transfer staff and three agency. Many of these nurses were afraid but many of them could not take their ugly beliefs, their racism, their hatred," Ashley explained.

"Did anyone stay?" Sura asked.

"A male nurse. A Viet Nam vet who saw lots of combat back then. And a young nurse. She's Mexican-American and has endured all of their nasty comments," Ashley said.

"Let me guess. She loves the challenge of caring for really sick patients and doing it well in spite of their beliefs," Sophia said.

"That's right, Sophia. I also understand she is able to take care of them by placing their beliefs in a box for the shift," Ashley said.

"There's a good amount of compartmentalizing involved in caring for populations you're not in agreement with all the time in terms of beliefs, values, world views, really.

"I mean when all of us look back to those years we did it also to a certain degree, didn't we?" Sophia concluded.

"You are right, Sophia. Our analyst. Sophia is a psychotherapist now, you know," Sura said to everyone at the table. "I sure didn't agree with our patients who were prostitutes and chose not to practice safe sex. I understood the money they needed to make in order to survive but not that."

Sura continued, "Remember Kimberly, Sophia and Cal. I put myself aside when I was with her. I practically forgot I even had that view. She felt like a daughter to me after all those months. Hardly anyone visited her and when they did they made her feel terrible about herself. I used to bring in German food for her that I made at home."

"That is exactly what we are talking about, Sura," Gerald said. "Most nurses and doctors, and I include myself, cannot do that for days or weeks, or even just for long shifts, with people who are so different from us."

Then Gerald emphasized, "We need nurses who can get close enough to these patients so we can find out what they have in common besides their awful racism."

Linda spoke now. "But why Gerald are you so concerned about this disease, or diseases, right now? The numbers are so low, comparatively speaking, to what we dealt with then. No one ever worked this fast for AIDS patients."

"I can only tell you that if I have an agreement from all of you to maintain the strictest confidentiality about what I'm about to say," Gerald said.

Everyone around the table said "Of course" or nodded their heads.

"Our first patient at the NHC with this new illness was admitted on May 17 with *Mycoplasma* pneumonia and quickly developed renal failure requiring dialysis."

"How is he now?" Bridgette spoke for the first time.

"His kidney function has improved on dialysis. But now he has these purple lesions on his torso, mainly. They are widening and deepening. They are somewhat painful but I am not sure of their significance beyond that. It's not good though," Gerald explained.

"How old is this one?" Dan asked now.

"21," Gerald said.

"So, this is your so-called patient zero?" Thomas asked.

"We never liked that term," Linda said.

"That's right," Sura said, and Sophia agreed.

"It blames one person for the whole lot of sufferers with any disease. And we bloody well know one person was not responsible for spreading around HIV, for fuck's sake," Jack said and added, "Sorry about that last bit."

"Oh my gosh," Ashley said. "It's like I've died and gone to liberal heaven."

"So, who is this young gentleman?" Cal asked. "He seems perdy dang important."

"Yeah, he sounds like the reason the other patients are there with him. Why else would men from Alabama and Georgia be at the NHC?" Sophia said.

"Ronnie Lynch, the Vice President of the United States' son," Gerald responded.

"Well, I'll be," Cal said.

"I hope he's not as big of a prick as his father," Fred said.

"We understand he falls in line with the other men on our unit," Ashley said.

Sophia said, "Let me get this straight. You want all of us to take care of these patients, the four men and now one woman..."

Ashley interrupted her. "And anyone else we get transferred to NHC with this disease."

"Until we can figure out the common source of the infections, hopefully leading to the discovery of this new virus," Sophia finished.

"That's right," Gerald said.

"That could take bloody months," Jack said.

"I, we, don't think so. We have some leads already. Some of the patients have mentioned pigs and white babies," Gerald said.

"And, oh, Gerald, we forgot the most important clue. Young Ronnie Lynch went to a bar down in Atlanta over this past Spring Break," Ashley added.

"How did you find out that?" Sophia asked.

"His Secret Service man saved a napkin and gave it to Ronnie's nurse at that time, Kristi," Ashley said.

"Very, very interesting. All of this. Well, I'm in. I'm back in the States for most of the summer anyway," Sophia said. "*But*, and it's a big but, I haven't practiced nursing since 1995, or '96," Sophia said.

"Me neither," Jack said.

"You still have licenses though?" Ashley asked them.

"Inactive," Sophia said and Jack said the same.

"We can take care of that ASAP," Ashley said.

"Is anyone else willing to help us?" Gerald asked.

All of the nurses said they were, including Sura and Linda who continued to talk to each other as the rest of the nurses talked to Ashley. They knew they were too old to work on the floor again but they wanted to stay.

"Ashley, I'm nearing 90 and Linda here is ...." Sura did not want to answer for her.

"I'm 81," Linda said.

"We can employ you two as consults, can't we Gerald?" Ashley said.

"Here's the great news. Well, not as great as having all of you here with us and willing to do some tough work once again.

"We have a good amount of money to pay all of you nicely, no matter what capacity you are willing to work in," Gerald said to all of them.

"How much is nicely?" Thomas Bechtel was the only one who asked.

"$150 per hour, or more if that's not enough," Gerald explained.

"Whooee!" Cal said. Me and Teddy can take that Alaskan cruise I've been talking about forever."

"Cal, keep in mind we may end up reliving some really bad stuff. These patients sound really sick, really challenging, like emotionally," Sophia said.

"But we'll all have each other," Cal said looking down at the floor.

JUNE 6, 2021, 4:00 P.M.
Crystal Nightingale Hotel Lounge, Crystal City, Va.

Sophia found Sura and Linda sitting in some red velvet chairs near the fireplace sipping what looked like bourbon on the rocks. She knew this fireplace would not house any wood until well into January, if at all. Sophia thought about the cold, frosty winters of her youth, now exchanged for tepid, wet ones, at best, by ailing Mother Nature.

Sophia checked into this hotel not long after leaving The Lincoln Hotel and then Terri at the train station. She thought about their conversation before approaching Sura and Linda.

"Soph, I don't know about this, about you staying here," Terri said.

Sophia did not say anything.

"I mean it looks like you are only just beginning to confront your past with AIDS. And now you've just signed up to be a nurse again for a bunch of really sick bigots," Terri continued.

"Well, at least they don't have AIDS," Sophia said.

"Does it matter? It's gonna kick up all that death stuff in you real fast."

"I think I may need to have all of it, or some of it, purged, Terri, if that's even possible. I don't know. But more importantly, I feel like I still have my desire to take care of sick patients."

"You do that as a therapist now."

"I know but I would like to see if I can still do it as a nurse. I always knew there was a reason I never gave up my license. Now I know."

"I love you, sis," Terri said and hugged Sophia. "My only solace is that you have Sura and Sura has Liz."

Sophia kissed her sister on the cheek and said, "Give one to Leslie and June. And to Ma, of course."

"She's gonna blow a fuse, Soph."

"I know. I'll call her tonight."

"Hello, Sophia," Sura said when Sophia reached the fireplace.

"Sit down with us, sweetie. Linda here was just telling me about how she ended up in San Francisco."

JANUARY, 1983
Navarro County, Texas

Linda always wanted to leave Texas, ever since she got there. Her mother moved them to Corsicana, to live with her auntie, when her father left them back in New Orleans. Linda's mother always said she was a handful. Linda liked to explore, and the wild streets of New Orleans where they lived until Linda was ten years old suited her personality.

When Linda met Paul Washington in nursing school in 1961, she knew he was the right man for her. He was kind, smart, and most importantly to Linda, he gave her room to breathe. She hoped after their honeymoon in San Francisco in 1965, he would want to settle there like Linda did.

But Paul loved Texas, a lot. He was born and raised in Corsicana. His grandfather, Toby, had been forced to work on the big corn plantation that supplied the grain for most of the eastern part of the state.

"Why, San Francisco, honey bunny?" Paul would always ask her. "All those hills will break a man's back."

"That's what those plantation owners did to your grand-daddy," Linda would always say. Linda took some pride in the fact that her family were free born Creoles in New Orleans. Most of them worked as servants in the swankiest hotels in the French Quarter.

"But they ain't done it to me, honey."

"Not in the same way, Paul. You've, we've, had to work much too hard to get to the same place white people begin at. Color doesn't mean quite as much out in San Francisco. I'd like to try it someday, soon," Linda would always say.

When Paul finished school after studying nights for years while working as an orderly in the hospital where Linda trained, he was offered a job as a lab technologist there. Linda stayed on in the ICU where she had been working since graduation.

The children they wanted never came naturally so they adopted a spunky five-year-old named Anthony in 1970. Then, Linda knew for sure they would not be going anywhere anytime too soon.

She just never imagined she would be leaving Texas the way she was now.

Paul had died right before the holidays. He was only 45 but his heart was much older. Linda asked Anthony to go with her. She knew he would love San Francisco. He was almost eighteen now and wanted to study fashion design. He applied to the art school in Dallas without telling Linda because he did not want to disappoint her if he did not get in.

Not only was Anthony accepted in the program, he was really in love with Charles, his best friend, for the past two years. Linda and Paul knew Charles had a much deeper place in Anthony's heart but never said a word about it to their son. They waited until he was ready to tell them.

Linda was scared for him, though. She saw how young men like her son were being treated. The ones who were getting sick and coming into the ICU with pneumonias and dying there alone had boyfriends who were banned from their bedsides by parents who did not understand.

Linda filled out her application for a nursing job at Bay City General Hospital in San Francisco on New Year's Day and mailed it out the following. She was hired as a float nurse by the end of the month.

She had no idea she would be landing in the West Coast's epicenter of an epidemic that was transforming young, beautiful men into wraiths.

JUNE 6, 2021, 4:00 P.M.
Crystal Nightingale Hotel Lounge, Crystal City, Va.

"It's so great you're here, Linda. I, we, always wanted to get out there and see what all of you did," Sophia said.

"I always wanted to come east, to see the differences, if there were any," Linda said.

"I wish you would've. We needed all the help we could get then dealing with the ugliness from everyone else. We were like the leper colony at Upper East Side Medical," Sophia explained.

"I know. It took us years to get Bay City beyond that," Linda said.

"I'm not sure we ever did," Sophia said and Sura nodded.

"Linda, how did you end up there? On the very first one?" Sura asked.

"It was ideal for me taking that float nurse position at Bay City General. I got to explore the hospital at work and the city during my time off.

"I kept seeing young men with wasting syndrome, crazy infections, and bowel disorders. They were so sick, and in so much danger," Linda explained.

"In the hospital or the streets of San Francisco?" Sura asked.

"Both. Then I heard about the unit opening and I wanted to take care of them, to keep them safe," Linda said.

"When I did the ER right out of nursing school I couldn't stomach the way they were treated," Sophia added.

"Sophia knows I worked on the oncology unit at Upper East Side Medical for years before our AIDS unit opened. They were always with us. I thought they should be, but almost everyone else I worked with did not feel that way at all," Sura said.

"I still remember my first one with Kaposi's Sarcoma. It was 1980 or '81," Sura said.

"That sounds about right," Linda said. "I was working ICU in Texas then. Charles was his name. He was so young and had been living in Dallas. His lungs were filled with it. When we extubated him after he died we saw one huge purple mass in the back of his throat. It's no wonder he couldn't breathe, even on the ventilator."

"You two make me feel so young. I wasn't even in nursing school then," Sophia said.

"Sophia, I knew you in the mid-80s. You were young in years maybe, but you have always been an old soul," Sura said.

"That's what Ricky always said too, Sura. He was my husband, Linda. He said if he lived to be one hundred, he still wouldn't have caught up with me," Sophia said.

"He was always right about you, Sophia."

"Anyway, Harry. Dr. Harry Greenberg," Sura continued. "He was older, a psychiatrist at Upper East Side Medical for years. Very respected. He had children, grandchildren. He had been widowed for years. The other nurses told me his wife died on our unit from colon cancer long before I started working there."

Sura then told them Harry's oncologist had been treating his KS for two years before she met him. Interferon injections were given in the office instead of admitting him to the oncology floor so no one knew. Dr. Greenberg was still practicing medicine then.

"I remember the night he was admitted. His KS was out of control. The oncology fellow on call, Max, I can't remember his surname, but I remember he was Chinese, thought he knew Harry from his residency days downtown.

"He told me when he returned to the nurse's station after examining Harry, 'That man. I never saw anything like it. The dermatologist, Dr. Harris, who performed the procedure then never did either."

Max told Sura Harry was referred to this dermatologist because he had pressure in his right ear. The ENT specialist could not find anything wrong inside his ear canal, but he had found a discolored lump behind the ear.

Sura repeated what Max said next. "'Dr. Harris found much more than a lump. When he excised it, Dr. Harris fell to the floor. I grabbed the forceps from his hand saving the purple golf-ball sized mass.'"

Sura then told them the pathology department could not determine the histology, the tissue type, of the mass so Max said Dr. Harris asked for some of it to be sent to the National Cancer Center. The pathologist there was able to conclude it was Kaposi's Sarcoma only because he had received tissue from an L.A. medical center one month before with the same diagnosis. These were the first two cases in the United States.

"As Linda knows all too well, it was strange back then seeing this type of cancer in young men who happened to be gay, or in older men like Harry Greenberg who were not.

"But as it turns out, Harry was. He had known that for a long time. He told me one night when I was changing his wet sheets after I irrigated his mouth with a peroxide solution I concocted to help clean away the blood oozing from his gums where the Kaposi's had eaten through."

Harry Greenberg was always faithful to his wife, Helen. He loved her. He knew she was an attractive woman, he just wasn't attracted to her. Their three children led to twice as many grandchildren. He never acted upon his desires until Helen died.

"Then he told me, he went a little crazy. That was 1975 when everyone was going crazy. He had been frequenting gentlemen's clubs in the West Village. But when the Studio opened in 1977, the lid on his restraint was blown straight off."

Sophia had to interrupt. "She means Studio 54, Linda. Anyone who ever got in called it the Studio."

Linda laughed. "We heard about it in San Francisco. Men I

took care of who spent any time in New York talked about it. So, Sura, how often did you go to the Studio?"

"Only once. I will not exaggerate. I was with my husband, Harold, and my friend Liz then, my wife now, who worked in the blood bank. It was a *heftig* night, as we say in German."

"Harry told me he went almost every night when the club first opened. I can't even imagine. One night of that kind of partying was enough to last me a lifetime."

Sura continued to tell them Harry said his children started to notice his new set of friends and his new interests. His oldest son, a neurologist, ran cognitive tests on him to see if early dementia could explain his behavior, and he was disappointed it could not.

"Harry stayed with us a long time. We gave him heavy duty chemotherapy. The more we gave, the sicker he got. No one in his family visited him. A friend came once. I could see they had been close but that young man looked sicker than Harry."

Sura told them the biggest disappointment, though, was the way the other nurses treated him. Only two other nurses would take care of Harry and even they said things to him.

"'You should've known better than that, Dr. Greenberg.'"

"'You should call your son and tell him you're sorry so he visits you.'"

Sophia responded. "I never understood how a nurse could blame a patient for his own illness. We are supposed to be the comforters."

"That was not easy to find back then, was it ladies?" Linda said.

"I still have not reached the worst part for Harry," Sura said.

"How much worse does it get, Sura?" Linda asked.

"I guess someone could have painted a red cross on his

bedroom door like they did centuries ago to homes in Europe when the plague visited," Sophia added.

"At least if that happened I could have still been his nurse. At least he would have had someone who touched him and spoke kind words to him," Sura said.

Sura explained the hospital administration at that time decided to move any patients with uncommon pneumonias, cancers, or weight loss to the uninsured wards. "That way the nicer beds would be available for patients with 'normal diseases,' as they were called."

"Indeed. I remember when I was floating at Bay City General, most of these men were placed on the indigent ward before our unit opened, even if they had insurance and money. Administration wanted them all hidden away," Linda added.

"Did you see Harry before he died? It's hard to believe you never told me about him, Sura" Sophia said.

"The last time I saw him was the night I transferred him. I still can't get it out of my mind. Maybe that's why I never mentioned him, Sophia. Plus, we had so many much worse off than him.

"He was yelling as I pushed his stretcher down the hallway. 'Why am I moving? For God's sake, Sura, I've been a doctor in this hospital for decades.'

"And when we put him into that dirty four-bedded room he cried out even louder, 'I'm a human being, my God. I am human.'

"He died two days later," Sura concluded.

Linda's head was lowered.

"Are you alright, dear?" Sura asked.

Linda's eyes were filled with tears that would not flow when she lifted up her head to answer Sura. "My son said the same thing when he was hospitalized with pneumonia."

"When was that, Linda?" Sophia asked.

"Back in '86. He had been living in Dallas after he graduated from design school. That's why he didn't come with me to San Francisco. Well, it was that but also Charles, his best friend, his lover, his partner," she said.

Linda told them she had seen Anthony over the Christmas holiday. He had been working at a major department store designing clothes but also buying. He traveled a lot, mainly to Hong Kong. That's why Linda thought he looked so thin.

"So how much weight have you lost, Anthony?" she could not help asking him.

"I don't know, Mother. Just a little. It's been hard. I love my job but I miss Charles," Anthony said.

She told them more. Linda and Anthony were sitting in the breakfast nook in Anthony's kitchen with a spectacular view of the city's skyline, hanging like a vibrant print outside the window, sipping chamomile tea and enjoying warm biscuits with drips of honey that Linda knew Anthony loved so much.

"Where is Charles, Anthony? It looks like he doesn't even live here."

"Well, he doesn't, Mother. We split about six months ago."

Linda could not help herself. She asked him if he had been careful.

"It's funny how I felt I could talk freely with young men in San Francisco I didn't know. But it was so different with my own son," she said to Sura and Sophia.

"I can only imagine," Sophia said and Sura agreed not having any children of her own either.

Linda continued to tell them how Anthony had begged Charles to stay, but Charles had been involved with an older man for a while. The man was married and went out to the bars almost every night. That's where Charles met him.

Charles felt protected with this man, though, and loved in a way Anthony could not provide. Charles wanted, needed, a strong, older man in his life. He lost his father right before he turned ten.

At twenty-one, Anthony could not even come close to filling up this emptiness in Charles. And this man did not either, in the end. He was hospitalized more often than not, Charles had told Anthony the last time he saw him when he came to collect the rest of his things, and Charles knew he was never going to leave his wife.

"I told Anthony he needed to be tested," Linda said to them. "I said I would go with him to the STD clinic in downtown Dallas before I flew back to San Francisco. I told him to call me anytime, day or night. I told him I loved him and he always had a home."

By the time Anthony received his positive results, he was really sick. His doctor told him about a new hospital for AIDS patients in Houston. He was admitted there. That's when he called Linda.

Linda had heard a little bit about The Hospital for Immune Diseases in Houston. She was impressed that Texas, the state she could not wait to leave, would have opened a hospital, a haven, for people with AIDS.

That was what she had thought before she arrived. It was more like a repository for the illest of the ill. Linda told Sura and Sophia it looked really nice, sparkly even, in that art deco sort of way that many American cities embraced in its architecture in the 1980s.

"It sure looked more appealing than our ward at Bay City General. And the location in Houston was much nicer than 12th and Folsom in San Francisco. But once you scratched the surface, that hospital was not serving those patients well at all."

Linda said Anthony's private room, they were all private, had not been cleaned in weeks. Dust balls rolled under the bed in sync with the door opening and closing, and imprints of over-active bowels decorated the toilet bowl.

"We know how terrible they all looked then. Sometimes I felt like I was rounding in a concentration camp barracks at Bay City General.

"But when I saw my boy, my Anthony. It had only been two months since I was in Dallas with him but my God! I only knew it was him in that bed when he opened his eyes. I could see the tiny grey flecks in his irises. I always called him starry night when he was a child."

"They sound beautiful, Linda," Sophia said.

"They were. But that skeleton lying there with his eyes was not my son.

"He started to cry when I hugged him and kissed him."

"Mother, I'm so glad you're here. It feels so good to be touched. I am human, you know. I need to be touched."

"Of course, you do, Anthony. Does anyone here help you, make you feel good?"

"Maria on nights. My Mexican Nightingale. She's a wonderful nurse."

Linda then told Sura and Sophia she called her director of nursing at Bay City General and asked for an immediate leave of absence.

She moved into his room.

Turn after turn, diaper after diaper, clean sheets after dirty ones, warm baths followed by lotion followed by cold compresses for the temperature spikes, toothette after toothette placed in his mouth so he could suck water from the pink sponge flavored with mint, and Motown tune after tune sung softly and smoothly by Linda carried Anthony out of this world almost two weeks later.

Right before he died he said, "Thank you, Mother."

"Please don't," Linda said. You are my son. I love you."

"Thank you for loving me."

"Those were his last words," Linda told them. "I was paralyzed sitting there holding his hand losing heat faster than I thought it would.

"I did not realize it then but all of my patients, the people I cared for during the three years before Anthony's death, were right there with me. It felt like one big mound that would not stop growing."

"Like the shoes," Sura said.

"Yes, like the shoes," Linda said. Sophia just kept nodding her head.

JUNE 6, 2021, 6:00 P.M.
Crystal Nightingale Hotel Lounge, Crystal City, Va.

Linda, Sura, and Sophia were ordering some dinner when Jack and Bridgette approached the bar and ordered some drinks.

"Top of the evening to you, ladies," Jack said. "You've met Bridgette here at the museum yesterday. She was like family to me once upon a time."

Bridgette smiled only to be polite and said, "He never really made it to that status."

SUMMER, 1986
East Village, New York City

Bridgette's sister, Fiona, moved here a year before. She was a painter. Struggling artists, even starving ones, could afford to live together, albeit in fifth floor walk-ups with no hot water.

Fiona met Jack at The Village Community Center in July while visiting a good friend, a sculptor, on Jack's unit. Their attraction was immediate and intense. After a month of dining in off beat restaurants, attending the funkiest art shows, and enjoying lots of steamy sex, Jack asked Fiona to move in with him.

Fiona cared about him, really, she loved Jack enough to introduce him to the rest of the Delaneys in Baltimore. Bridgette really got to know him when she moved to the Village, too. It was the only place she felt like she could be herself.

The Delaney family in Baltimore, Maryland, boasted two priests and three nuns, and that was only since they came to the U.S.A. in 1917 from County Galway in Ireland. Bridgette almost made number four. That was until 1985 when she started to realize she might have entered the convent at St. Patrick's on Calvert Street to avoid facing what she always knew.

By the time she made novitiate, serving in the convent community for two years already and earning the title "Sister," she was involved with Catherine, a canonical novitiate in her last stage of preparing to take permanent vows for a life to serve Jesus Christ and the Catholic Church while supposedly being celibate.

Bridgette asked her to leave the nunnery with her, but Catherine could not do it. She had no other training and she could never imagine living her life openly as a lesbian. Bridgette was a little more fortunate. She was trained as a nurse. She had attended The Hebrew Hospital for the Poor Nursing School before she entered the convent.

Bridgette would always be known as the "failed nun" in her family, the Church, and the Irish community. Only The Hebrew Hospital did not care about all of that so she returned to working there as an RN after she left the convent. But it turned out everyone cared about her being a lesbian.

Bridgette started working with Jack at Village Community

right as her sister and him split up.

June 6, 2021, 6:00 P.M.
Crystal Nightingale Hotel Lounge, Crystal City, Va.

"I should've been though. I wish I had," Jack responded to Bridgette's comment about him not being family while inhaling a shot of Jameson's whiskey. "Christ knows, it's taken me the better part of me life to mend the broken pieces of me heart."

Jack Doherty always thought they split because Fiona was not happy with the long night shifts he worked at the hospital. But Bridgette knew her sister was not happy with the long nights Jack spent at the pub when he was off duty.

"Hey, isn't it amazing the way NHC has arranged for all of this?" Sophia tried to steer the subject away from maudlin indulgences in failed romances.

"Well then, Sophia, we are doing them a bit of a favor, aren't we?" Jack quipped back.

"I suppose we are, Jack, but we are being compensated nicely," Sura said.

"Sura and I aren't even going to be physically taking care of them up there," Linda said pointing to the hospital that could be seen through the floor to ceiling window they had been sitting next to ever since they decided to order dinner here.

Bridgette added, "I couldn't agree more. I was only planning on being in D.C for a week, but this is one great opportunity provided by the hospital, the government, or the Vice President of the United States himself taking care of all of our expenses. I bet he would shit a brick if he knew some of us were gay."

Everyone laughed.

Jack said, "The ladies are always right to be sure." Then he ordered a glass of water at the bar.

"Does anyone know where the rest of us are tonight?" Sophia asked.

"I saw Cali and Teddy catching a taxi to the airport," Jack said as he returned to the table.

"Oh, that's right, Teddy kept his flight back to San Francisco," Sophia said.

"Cali told Teddy I would keep an eye on her while we worked here. I assured Teddy of me good intentions. Teddy said, 'It's not you, Jack, I'm worried about.' Then he hugged me goodbye."

"I imagine Fred is saying goodbye to Li at the airport, too. He came with him to see the Quilt," Linda said.

"So, who does that leave?" Sophia asked.

"The tall one. Thom, I think. Does anyone know him?" Sura asked.

Everyone said they did not.

"Oh, and that Italian-American man," Sophia added.

"That's Danny, Dan," Linda said. "He has a good heart. No bitterness in it in spite of all the defeats he's had over the years. He lived in L.A. a long time, but I'm pretty sure he came back east not too long ago."

"So, Jack, I guess we're the only two who need a refresher course," Sophia said.

"We're real slackers, to be sure," Jack said and smiled.

"What's so amazing to me is how quickly Ashley made it happen. I mean just one course tomorrow and we're back on duty again," Sophia said.

"That's power working, for us, for a change. I'll tell you I went inactive a few years ago, when I cared for Mom back home in Baltimore. When I wanted to work again it took about three months of class time and clinical hours to reactivate my license," Bridgette explained.

"Wow, Bridgette. You're not kidding. Hey, what kind of nursing do you do now?" Sophia asked.

"Hospice. Home Hospice. I never left Baltimore after Mom died in 2015. I've actually grown to like the city. It's caught up with New York in many ways," Bridgette said.

"That's admirable what you do," Sura added.

"I think I can really see how our AIDS patients back then, in the beginning of my career, prepared me for it now, at the end of it," Bridgette said.

"It was never official that's what we were doing then, was it?" Sophia said. "I mean the doctors, at least the infectious disease ones and especially the oncologists, kept treating them like they would get better. But we knew."

Everyone nodded.

The food arrived. Poached salmon with a light Hollandaise sauce and jasmine rice for Sophia, beef Wellington for Sura, and Liz who had joined them now after a long nap in their room, and pork tacos with black beans for Linda.

Jack asked Bridgette if she wanted to have some dinner at an Irish pub he found a few blocks away. But before they left, Jack asked Sophia if she would like to meet "for a wee breakfast in the morn" prior to their training.

"I'd love too, Jack. How about right here around 0700?" Sophia said.

"It's a date, love. See you then," Jack said as he and Bridgette said goodbye to the table.

As the ladies were enjoying one shot espressos after dinner, Dan Napolina entered the lounge in search of a nightcap.

"Hello, Danny. Come sit with us," Linda said. "Where did you eat tonight?"

"I found a pizzeria a few blocks over. The manicotti was pretty good, so was the Chianti. But I'm still so wired, jacked up by what we're about to do. I thought a Sambuca or a Bailey's might help carry me off to la la land. I always like to have a good night's rest before first shift," Dan said.

"It's nice to meet you again, Dan," Sophia said. Sura said the same and introduced him to Liz. Dan returned the sentiments.

"Where do you work now?" Sophia asked. "I'm assuming you do because you do not need a refresher."

"I moved back to Jersey a few years ago. From LA. My fadder had a stroke. I took care of 'em until he died last year. I do some agency there and back in L.A. whenever I'm in town," Dan replied.

Sophia was thinking how much he sounded like her brother, Diego. She used to think the Bronx and New Jersey were worlds away.

Dan continued, "I have to. I never made the money I thought I would with my screenplays. Forget about the acting."

"You write screenplays? What are they about?" Sophia asked.

"That's a story for another time," Dan said. "I'm just so glad our licenses are national now, no need for state ones like in the old days."

"Who is on with you tomorrow?" Sura asked.

"That tall guy. What's his name again?" Dan asked.

"Thom, we're told," Linda said. "You don't know him at all, Danny?"

"Nah, never met him. I guess I will tomorrow. Ashley said she thought some male nurses should start first, to set the tone for the patients up there," Dan said.

"It sounds like Ashley Smith may be young in years but wise in her decisions," Sophia said.

"That sounds a little familiar doesn't it, Sophia?" Sura said while hugging her.

JUNE 7, 2021, 1:00 P.M
National Health Center, Respiratory Unit, Staff Lounge

"What the hell's wrong with these guys, Tommy?" Dan said to Thomas as they sat down for a lunch break, not a regular occurrence on any nursing unit but Ashley Smith provided coverage for them by floating nurses from a less busy floor. She really did not want to lose any of them before more clues were found for this new disease's cause.

"I believe, Daniel, my experience today, thus far, has been quite different than yours," Thomas said.

"Yeah, no shit. You could pass for one of 'em, though. I'm assuming you're not, considering you were an AIDS nurse back in the day like the rest of us here now."

"You would be correct, Daniel."

"So why the hell do ya talk like that, as if you're British fuck'n royalty or sometin."

"Forgive my formalities. I've never been able to shake, so to speak, my heritage."

"Where you from Tommy boy?"

"Philadelphia."

"I'm assuming not South Phili."

"Right, more like Rittenhouse Square."

"Oh, I get it. You're rich. How come you're a nurse then?"

FALL, 1984
Ben Franklin Hospital, Philadelphia

Thomas Bechtel was in his last year of medical school applying for residencies ultimately leading to a cardiology fellowship, just like his father expected. He was also expected to marry Jane Clark, a handsome woman from Old Main Line who had

recently completed her Bachelor's degree in German Literature and was waiting patiently for Thomas to ask for her hand.

But Thomas was in a rotation in Infectious Diseases and he
was not supposed to like it as much as he did. And he certainly
was not supposed to like the partner of one of his patients,
dying from Burkitt's lymphoma, as much as he did.

At first, Thomas thought he was just helping Peter cope
with Jonathan's AIDS-related cancer over lunches in the
hospital cafeteria. And then he thought he was just interested
in Peter's life because it was so much more interesting than
his own.

Peter was an art dealer specializing in paintings from the
Schuylkill River School of painters. Peter educated Thomas
about this school's influence on the much more famous Hudson
River School, but not credited as their influential antecedents.

Peter knew Old Main Line collectors who, from time to
time, wanted to set free one of their paintings for a museum or a
private sale. That's when Peter stepped in. His degree in Art
History provided him with the lens to spot a forgery in a
haystack, or to procure a small fortune for the most valuable
ones.

After Jonathan died, Thomas and Peter's lunches turned
into dinners, art auctions, and much less time spent with Jane.
Thomas also realized he did not want to practice medicine, but
he did want to help the really ill patients he met during his ID
rotation, the ones who no one else wanted to touch.

He told his parents he would finish medical school in the
Spring and then he was going to enroll in The Ben Franklin
School of Nursing, one of the oldest three-year diploma
programs in the country.

Thomas Bechtel was promptly disinherited. The wedding
to Jane was called off. Peter was the one now who splurged for
their dinners throughout Thomas' time in nursing school until

he died from Kaposi's Sarcoma in the summer of 1988, just in time for Thomas' graduation.

Thomas never did introduce Peter to his parents who he only visited during the Christmas holidays anyway. They never did know how much Thomas loved Peter. They never did know how careful he had been to have escaped infection with the virus.

JUNE 7, 2021, 1:05 P.M.
National Health Center, Respiratory Unit, Staff Lounge

"I began work on the AIDS Unit at Ben Franklin Hospital when I graduated in 1988, Daniel," Thomas told him.

"Look, ya gotta call me Dan, or Danny. Only my grandmother called me that, and only until I was like thirteen."

"My parents were not happy with my decision to not be a doctor and to not marry the woman they chose for me."

"I get it now, Tommy."

"Please, Dan, can you call me Thomas, or Thom is fine. Tommy is just a bit too juvenile for my taste."

"Yeah, there ain't too much juvey about you, heh. So how long did you work with AIDS patients?"

Thomas told him he left the unit in 1995 with the antiretroviral revolution, and then went on to become a nurse practitioner. He has been working in a Sexually Transmitted Disease clinic in Philadelphia ever since.

"And Dan, how long did you work with them?" Thomas asked as Margarita came into the breakroom for a quick bite to eat. She did not know what to do with herself for longer than fifteen minutes off the floor.

"I've always wanted to work with them. Oh, I am sorry to interrupt," she said.

"Don't be ridiculous, Margarita. Sit down and talk for a few," Dan said.

"I know from what I've read it was like a new discovery every day, all the diseases the virus caused."

"It was indeed," Thomas said. "Dan, do you remember when we figured out HIV crossed the blood brain barrier and produced those plaques along the neurons?"

Dan said, "Yeah, I remember. PML. Progressive Multifocal Leukoencephalopathy it was named, Margarita. It made 'em crazy if the virus went that way. I particularly remember a guy I took care of for a minute."

"Where was that, Dan?" Thom asked.

"Westwood Community Central Hospital in L.A. Sanchez was his name. All of a sudden as his PCP was resolving, he started to scream every time any of us came near him. He looked terrified. I think he really was, the poor thing.

"But then he kept on screaming even after we left his room. That was like in 1990. That's when I remember the docs starting to write down the diagnosis in their charts."

Thomas nodded his head.

"So, what happened to Mr. Sanchez?" Margarita asked. "I know it wasn't good but did he get any relief in the end?"

"Not really. He screamed non-stop, day and night, and hit a few of us. But he didn't know what the hell he was doing.

"He had a wife and some kids but they couldn't take the noise. The wife was also sore at him for giving her the virus. That's the way she saw it. We always told her he didn't know he had HIV when they slept together before he got real sick.

"We tried everything on Sanchez, to calm him down. Steroids. Haldol. We knew when his room got real quiet it was only because he was real dead."

"That poor man," Margarita said with tears in her eyes.

"Hard to believe but he sounds nicer than most of our patients here."

"You betcha, Margarita. I've been takin care of George Johnson and he's mean as a snake," Dan said.

"Not if you're white," Margarita said.

"Well, that's just it. I always thought I was, but he called me a 'half-breed.' And that Sawyer guy called me a 'dego'. Only my grandfather was called that after he came through Ellis Island from Italy, like in 1920.

"In the end, though, I don't give a shit what they call me. I'm their nurse and they're sick. And Johnson is really sick with pneumonia, plus his kidneys are starting to shut down."

"That's interesting, Dan. Almost everyone with kidney failure has that purple rash," Margarita said. "I know Mr. Johnson has it."

"Mr. Lynch does, as well," Thomas said.

"I guess these patients here now really do have interesting illnesses, but their racism is just so horrible," Margarita said. "I try and place all of it in my imaginary box for the shift so I can take care of them."

"Yeah, it's funny, Margarita. I forgot until now how much we needed to do something with some of the stuff we saw back then. Granted, we weren't dealing with racist assholes so much, but, shit, I took care of people pimping whatever they could out on Sunset Boulevard at night and then landing on our AIDS Unit by day. We put ourselves aside, though, and just took care of 'em.

"Hey, Margarita, can you lend me the biggest box you got?" Dan asked.

Margarita laughed while pretending to hand him one.

JUNE 7, 2021, 6:30 P.M.
National Health Center, Respiratory Unit, Staff Lounge

After the lunch break, Margarita thought she could get used to every day, she prepared for another female patient being admitted with terrible diarrhea and early stage kidney failure from Atlanta Central Medical Center. Margarita also was taking care of Reba Smith who she assumed felt pretty sick because she did not insult the young nurse with any comments about the color of her skin.

The Atlanta doctor attributed Betty Ann Williams' kidney malfunction to the diarrhea but did not find any bacterial or other source for it so he reported her case to the CDB hotline last evening. And then Dr. Jack Durante called Dr. Gerald Brugge right before he went off duty this morning.

Mrs. Williams arrived via Medevac helicopter around 5:00 P.M. and Margarita worked as fast as she could to perform the nursing part of the admission because she knew Dr. Brugge was coming in earlier than his usual shift time.

Gerald entered the nurse's lounge now to share some information he obtained during the History and Physical he just finished performing in the patient's room.

"Margarita, did Betty Ann Williams say anything to you about her husband?"

"She said he's coming to visit her on Wednesday, that was the earliest he could get some time off from his job in Jackson, Georgia. I guess that's south of Atlanta," Margarita said.

"It is. Did she talk to you about any travel?"

"I asked her if she's been anywhere outside of the United States, or even Georgia, and she said she hasn't been."

Gerald said he had asked the patient the same questions, and then asked if her husband had been sick with diarrhea like she has been or anything else. "She said he has not been."

"Yes, Dr. Brugge I asked her that, too."

Gerald continued, "And then I asked her if her husband has traveled anywhere recently, even outside of Jackson in like the past six months."

"I didn't think to ask her that, doctor, after she said her husband hadn't been sick."

"She told me he went to Atlanta sometime in March. And I asked her if it was for some business of his. She said he met up with some friends who all do charity work together. Then I asked her what kind of work."

"She said for albino children. Isn't that what Tina said Mrs. Smith told her about Sam also?"

"Yeah, but I'm pretty sure Mrs. Smith told Tina the men who did that work also wore hoods, to feel what it's like to be blind," Margarita said.

"We might be getting somewhere," Gerald said as the other nurses started pouring into the room for shift report.

JUNE 8, 2021, 3:00 A.M.
National Health Center, Respiratory Unit

Bridgette Delaney did her rounds on Buddy Miller. She knew he was being discharged in the morning, if his diarrhea continued to stay under control. He walked out of the bathroom while Bridgette neatened his sheets. She just had set a fresh pitcher of water on his bedside table.

"You know, Mr. Miller, you need to continue drinking at least two liters of water a day, to stay hydrated."

"How much is that exactly? Give it to me in soda bottles."

"About one big one, 64 ounces, but no soda for you. Only water and juices."

"I would've been back home a week ago with a nurse like you."

"I understand you've had quite a few good nurses, some very experienced ones."

"I mean white ones," the patient said.

"What does color have to do with what's in here and here, Mr. Miller?" Bridgette pointed to her heart and head as she said it.

He said nothing. Then a few seconds later, "You know my wife left me for a Mexican."

"Maybe she did not leave because he's Mexican," Bridgette said.

"We were married twenty years, just about."

"Maybe there was something she wasn't happy about with herself or maybe in her relationship with you," Bridgette said as she tucked the sheets in around him to protect him from the strong air conditioning blowing in the room.

"She did mention, more than once, that I spent too much time doing my charity work."

"What kind of work do you do, Mr. Miller?"

"Helping blind children."

"That's a good cause. Now you best get some rest before we send you back to Georgia in the morning."

June 8, 2021, 5:00 A.M.
National Health Center, Respiratory Unit, Staff Lounge

"Hey FNG, how'd all of you princesses manage to get us regular breaks during our shifts?" Charlie said to Bridgette while thankful to sit down.

"We should always have a break. Only difference now is

Ashley is making sure we FNGs get them while we place our own lives on hold to help out the NHC here."

"You don't look old enough to have served," Charlie said.

"I'm not, but my brother did. He wrote letters every week. I picked up on their lingo," Bridgette said.

"Was he in country?"

"Yes. In '68."

1969–1970
Viet Nam

Charles Brown had been drafted not long after his eighteenth birthday in January, 1968. He was surprised how long it took to get deployed and thought about going to Canada but could not bring himself to do it.

He was in Viet Nam the following January at the newly built Firebase Crook, ready to get busy as the medic he was trained to be.

Marching into Cambodia did not take that long when the storm started. Charlie patched up the men's wounds and shot them out of their misery with all of the morphine injectables he collected from the fallen boys' bags of U.S.-issued goodies.

By the time he completed his unofficial tour in Cambodia, Charlie was pleased to have his life and his limbs. But those gifts were exchanged for thick layers of scars only allowing him to feel the faintest pricks of pain when someone he loved died, like his mother a decade after he came home, or left him, like his three wives over the next two decades; affection for the German shepherds he always had by his side; and to play in his mind over and over again, like a film reel rewinding to one scene, Will from Atlanta, who he spent 48 hours with in a foxhole until they received the all clear, whose shattered skull with his left eye still intact landed in his arms, and Sal from Brooklyn, from that same hole, whose right arm he carried to safety because he did not know what else to do with it except to remove Sal's high school ring he still wore on a chain around his neck to this day.

JUNE 8, 2021, 5:10 A.M.
National Health Center, Respiratory Unit, Staff Lounge

Charlie asked Bridgette, "Did he make it home OK, your brother?"

"Depends on if you view a body bag as OK. Personally, I'd say yes, considering what he had to do over there."

"I should've known better than to think I could ruffle your feathers. I forget the closest thing to an old Viet Nam vet is an old AIDS nurse," Charlie said.

"Guess it's all the dead we've been carrying around all these years," Bridgette said.

"Just don't stop because then you have to really think about it," Charlie said.

"So, Charlie, have you taken care of Miller before?" Bridgette did not want to go any deeper with him.

"I've met him a few times, but never for a whole shift."

Bridgette told him about her conversation with this patient earlier.

"That's something, isn't it. I've been taking care of George Johnson ever since Sam Smith died last weekend. His wife is there with him all the time and she's mentioned that same charity. She said, 'Georgie's real sad he can't be helping those blind children.'"

"Did you get the name of the charity, Charlie?"

"She didn't tell me. Tina, one of our regulars who talked a

lot with Mrs. Smith when Sam was still alive, said this charity was an excuse to be a Klansman."

"No shit. Like KKK, right? Ashley and Brugge had mentioned that to us last Saturday night."

"I wouldn't be a damned bit surprised with what I've heard the other nurses say. Personally, I haven't heard too much, mainly because I've been taking care of Smith on the ventilator since I've been here. That's the way I like them. Quiet."

"Where do you usually work, Charlie?"

"Surgical ICU. I'm looking forward to getting on back there too. Not ashamed to say."

"Well, I better get back out there. Thanks for the chat, Charlie," Bridgette said while Charlie just sat there staring at the floor.

JUNE 8, 2021, 7:30 A.M.
National Health Center, Respiratory Unit

Bridgette finished giving report. She had promised Buddy Miller she would wheel him downstairs to the car waiting at the main entrance.

The elevator door opened to a thin man sitting in a wheelchair accompanied by two paramedics, one holding his IV bag up high.

"Buddy, what you doing here?" the thin man said.

"Jimmy?" Buddy had a hard time recognizing him.

The thin man nodded his head and Buddy said, "I've been here a little while, but I'm going home today."

"What did you have, Buddy?"

"Diarrhea mainly, and some pneumonia. How about you?"

"Well, I've been in Atlanta General for about a week with diarrhea, too. Now they tell me my kidneys aren't so good and I needed to come all the way up here to figure out what's wrong with me."

"Well, I got better, Jimmy. You will too. Hang in there."

Bridgette wheeled Buddy onto the elevator and turned his chair around to face the door. "If you're lucky, you'll have this angel of mercy here. The *right* kind of nurse," Buddy added and winked before the door closed.

Outside, Bridgette opened the car door, but before she helped Buddy stand she asked him how he knew the man who came up to the floor on the elevator.

"We do some work together," Buddy said.

"Charity work?"

Buddy nodded and then stood up and kissed her on the cheek. "Thanks for taking such good care of me. Keep our race going, honey," he said and got in the back seat of the car.

Bridgette was only able to work up a smile for Buddy because all she could think of was if he only knew he just kissed a woman whose Black wife, Sandra, was waiting for her back home in Baltimore, he would shit.

Bridgette hurried back upstairs looking for Dr. Brugge. She found him getting ready to go into the new patient's room to perform a History and Physical his young ID fellow would help to complete before Gerald went off duty a little later than usual.

"Gerald, may I have a minute?"

"As long as you'd like, Bridgette," he said and they walked to the nearby on-call room for some privacy.

"That man in the room you're going into, Buddy Miller and I just met him coming up on the elevator. His name is Jimmy."

"That's right. James Wilson from Clayton, Georgia, where Miller is from, too. He was the one I told all of you about earlier in the night. He came from Atlanta Central Medical with diarrhea, renal failure, and some purple lesions."

"Well, they know each other," Bridgette said.

"How?" Gerald asked.

"Charity work."

"Our biggest clue so far."

"You mean besides their awful racism," Bridgette said.

"That's right, Bridgette."

Bridgette looked for Dan Napolina, James Wilson's assigned day shift nurse. He was outside of George Johnson's room. She told him the discharged Buddy Miller knew his new patient through charity work back home in Georgia.

"What kinda charity is that, like dry cleaning the Klan's hoods?" he said. "But thanks for the info, Bridgette, have a good rest."

JUNE 8, 2021, 3:00 P.M.
National Health Center, Respiratory Unit

So far, it had not been a good shift.

George Johnson went for a bronchoscopy in the morning and now was on a ventilator. *PCP* pneumonia was the diagnosis, just like Sam Smith a week before.

Ashley Smith was on the unit now making sure an ICU nurse could care for Mr. Johnson as the breathing machine was rolled into his room while the respiratory therapist squeezed oxygen into the patient's lungs through the ambu bag attached to the tube in his throat.

Dan did not wish for George Johnson to be in respiratory failure, but he was not disappointed the patient would not be able to speak. Earlier in the day, before the bronchoscopy, Dan was changing Mr. Johnson's central line dressing, administering the antibiotic followed by hanging a fresh bag of IV fluids, then draining the urine from the bag connected to the catheter in his bladder to measure how well his kidneys were still functioning when Mr. Johnson told him through labored breaths, "You seem to really know what you're doing for a dego."

"And you seem like you haven't lost your appetite, Mr. Johnson, for finding the nicest things to say to me," Dan replied.

Mrs. Johnson assured Dan her husband was just grumpy due to being hospitalized for too long and too often over the past couple of months. "You're very kind, Danny. I've been telling my friends back home my husband's nurse looks like a movie star, like that Al Pac.... I can't really pronounce it but he was in those older mobster movies."

MAY, 1982
Hollywood, California

Dan Napolina always wanted to be an actor, and technically he was. He trained at the Strasberg School in New York City in the mid-1970s. At least it got him out of Jersey and a little removed from his parents, three older brothers and three younger sisters.

He did get smaller parts in off, off Broadway plays, but everyone told him he would do so much better in L.A. He had that "Pacino look," they always told him.

Hollywood turned out to be seedier than Dan ever could have imagined, but it was easier to get work. At least he could pay his weekly rent on the room in the hotel off Sunset Boulevard and buy enough food to keep up a healthy appearance.

But even these amenities were only to be had if he accepted parts in skin flicks in which he had no choice acting with women or men. He pretended to be in someone else's body when he had to be with the men.

He thought he got his big break in 1979 when he landed

the role of the brother in a show about an Italian-American family struggling to make it out of the Bronx called *The Amicis on Arthur Avenue*. It never made it out of pilot.

Mrs. Napolina bragged to everyone about her son, the great actor, the next Pacino for sure. When Dan received the news about the show, he called her first.

"The show's not being picked up, Ma."

"I am so sorry, Danny. It's not you. You're a good actor. I've seen you in all your plays. But you should think about doin sometin else to keep yourself goin until you make it. You were always good in school, in science class."

"Ya, know Ma, I've been thinkin just that. I need more than this. I can't imagine being in this shitty room five years from now."

"So, what are you thinkin, Danny?"

"Nursing, Ma."

"I wouldn't of thought that, but you have a good heart and a good head."

"Well, like you say, I was always good in science and I really do give a shit about people. I don't even mind blood. They want more guys now, too, in the profession."

Dan payed his way through nursing school at Westwood Community Central's diploma program with the money he received from the failed pilot and was graduating now.

He had to let the acting go during school but planned on picking it up again after he passed his boards. He had a job offer at Westwood Community on the ward where he would meet plenty of fellow actors, including one of the most famous ones from films in the 1950s and 1960s where he pretended to be the love interest of some of the most beautiful actresses on and off screen.

June 8, 2021, 6:30 P.M.
National Health Center, Respiratory Unit, Staff Lounge

Dan was finishing up his charting on one of the portable pads the NHC supplied nurses with so they never had to be chained to a computer away from patients when Ashley Smith came in to check on him.

"I know you've had a rough day, Dan. I've arranged for ICU nurses to care for Mr. Johnson around the clock as long as he is ventilated. I know most staff nurses do not have any ventilator experience. I sure didn't."

"Ya know, Ash, we did back in the day out on the floor because the ICU nurses wouldn't touch 'em."

"You mean your AIDS patients?"

"I do. So we all learned real fast."

"You were in L.A. then, right?"

"I was, at Westwood. I thought about leaving when I graduated in '82, but so many of the people I worked with before then kept getting admitted."

"What did you do before nursing school, Dan?"

"I acted. Well, not successfully, not financially anyway."

"I remember watching an old movie with my mother once when I was a kid. It starred that handsome Rock Hudson. Then my mother told me he died from AIDS. I read everything I could about him, his movies, his life. It was so sad," Ashley said.

"Yeah, he didn't have it so good in the end."

"You took care of him?" Ashley's eyes widened.

Dan nodded, and then said, "Ya know, Ash, I've been working on Mrs. Johnson, ever since her husband got sedated on the ventilator."

"That's good."

"Yeah, I'm using my acting history as leverage. She thinks I'm like Al fuck'n Pacino or something."

Ashley laughed. "You do look like him, but much younger."

"You're kind. Anyway, we got to talkin about where they live down in Georgia, not too far from Savannah. I asked her if she and Georgie go there sometimes, to have some fun, ya know.

"So, she says they really don't go anywhere but Georgie does sometimes, usually around Halloween. So I asked her where."

"What did she say?"

"To North Carolina for Christmas pigs. I said to eat them? Then she says Georgie gets 'em for that, for them, but really for the blind children's charity. I asked her what charity but she didn't know the name but it's for albino kids," Dan said.

"My goodness, pigs and white children again," Ashley said.

"OK, so I says to her, 'how was the pork dinner on Christmas.'"

"What did she say, Dan?"

"She said they couldn't have it because the pig was too sick. So, I asked her what happened and she said the poor thing was real thin and looked weird, so I asked her weird how? And she said the pig looked kind of purplish."

"Like her husband now," Ashley said.

"That's right. Then I says to her, 'so the pig died, right?' And she told me Georgie took care of 'em."

Then Charlie came in. Ashley told him his only patient would be Mr. Johnson tonight since he was ventilated. Charlie was happy to have a quiet one again.

And then Sophia opened the door and said, "Report room, right?"

"Hi, Sophia," Ashley said. "How was your refresher course yesterday?"

"Intense, but good. All of the technology now is a little scary."

"Don't worry, Charlie is on tonight," Ashley said and introduced them to each other. "Plus, we have a floating IT nurse, we have to with all of the agency nurses we use. We don't want the computers coming between the patient and the nurse."

"It's OK if they do sometimes," Charlie said. "Nice to meet you, Sophia." And then he mumbled to himself, "another FNG."

"What does that mean, Dan?" Sophia said in Dan's ear while Charlie talked with Ashley about his differential ICU pay for this shift.

"The nurses I worked with in L.A. who served in Nam used to say it. It means 'Fuck'n New Guy.' That's what they said when a new soldier came into the field with them."

Charlie was now pouring a cup of coffee.

"Nice to meet you too, Charlie. I wish I was a FNG but really I'm a FOG," Sophia said.

"This is gonna be fun after all," Charlie said as Jack Doherty entered the breakroom.

JUNE 9, 2021, 3:00 A.M.
National Health Center, Respiratory Unit

"Honey, you've been so good to me all night. And patient," Betty Ann Williams said to Sophia as she turned her again to clean her and change her sheets.

"Where are you from, Nurse? You look so exotic."

"I'm from New York, Mrs. Williams. Call me Sophia."

"Well, you could've fooled me. I thought you were from somewhere far away like Arabia or Persia."

"No, Ma'am, just New York," Sophia said while hanging her next IV bag of Normal Saline with Potassium, recording the volume of the empty bag she took down and the urine she just emptied from her catheter bag.

"How's my urine looking, Nurse Sophia?"

"Fine. We would like to see more of it but it's fine for now."

"I'm more concerned right now, honey, about this rash. I'm not really sure what it is, down near my privates."

"May I take a look, Mrs. Williams?"

"Sure enough. You are my nurse. I haven't let that male one see it, even if he is right handsome. Exotic looking, too, like you."

Sophia knew the patient was talking about Dan Napolina. Sophia thought it was funny how back home in the northeast or in Italy, everyone was "exotic looking" as she lit the lower end of the long light over the patient's bed, lifted her sheets, and examined her lower abdominal area. She found two large purplish lesions growing into each other in an irregular pattern.

"I'm glad you showed me, Mrs. Williams. You get some rest now," Sophia said as she covered her with the blanket and turned off the light.

Sophia took off her gown and gloves and washed her hands in the anteroom. She stepped into the dark hallway that had a saucy reddish hue from the night lights lining the top of the walls.

And then Sophia drifted back to the summer of 1988.

He was sitting up fixing his face in the mirror nestled in the bedside table that crossed over the bed.

"Sophia Loren, darling, come to me, please. Tell me what you see." He always called her that and Sophia always fibbed to him every time he placed this request.

"I see the most beautiful man, Reynaldo. The talk of the town, the envy of every other man whose arm you're not holding onto in your body-sculpted-sequined pants suit, strutting your stuff in those white leather platform shoes walking into the hottest clubs in Sao Paulo."

And then he would always give Sophia a regretful smile, and sigh, "If only I had stayed away from the Studio and those Lower West Side clubs, I would not have to make up my face like this now."

Reynaldo had confided in Sophia after only knowing her a few nights. He had been a prostitute when he came to New York from Brazil, sometimes frolicking with a dozen or more partners a night. But he made a lot of money. He had a steady older lover, Sven, from Copenhagen, with whom he lived for a while.

That was before Sven got sick and his wife back home started calling him a faggot and Sven started beating Reynaldo. So, when the Kaposi's Sarcoma started popping up on Reynaldo's face he initially thought Sven's bruises were just fading slower than usual.

After Sven died, Reynaldo was on the streets, trying to turn enough tricks to just buy a meal and pay for his room without running water above one of the Times Square theatres where he heard sordid noises coming from the film playing that he remembered coming from the rooms he once hustled.

All the men stopped wanting him when he could no longer conceal the cancer on his face or his waifish figure. Then Reynaldo had to make any empty storefront, that didn't kick him away, his home for the night.

Sophia was on duty the night he was admitted. Scabies embedded the surface of his skin, skipping his face, as if the little mites were above visiting the cancer.

"Tell me, darling, Sophia Loren," she heard him so clearly now standing in the dark, "Am I not still so beautiful?"

"Gorgeous, Reynaldo," she said.

"Thank you, Sophia Loren."

Before Sophia turned to walk away she saw one tear rolling down his cheek interrupting the smooth surface of his makeup and revealing the tips of large purple masses buried beneath. And she heard him say, "She's so right. I still have it."

June 9, 2021, 3:30 A.M.
National Health Center, Respiratory Unit

Ronnie Lynch's pneumonia had resolved, his diarrhea was almost gone, his required daily fluid balance was more or less controlled and calculated by the dialysis nurses, yet tonight Sophia felt he was much more challenging to take care of than Betty Ann Williams.

Ronnie had been emotional lately, according to Thomas Bechtel who gave Sophia report earlier. Why wouldn't he be? Sophia thought entering his room now. He's a boy without a diagnosis or a discharge date.

When Sophia introduced herself to Ronnie at the beginning of the shift, he asked her, "So how long have you been legal?"

"Whatever do you mean, Ronnie? Sophia responded.

"How did you get across the border?"

"Do you mean the Italian border where I've lived for some time now as a permanent American resident?"

"Oh, when did you become a citizen here?"

"When I was born in New York in 1965," Sophia said.

"Wow, I pegged you for a Mexican, maybe Salvadoran."

"And I pegged you for a young man who hasn't had the opportunity to experience the world outside the confines of his own family."

Ronnie did not say much after that except to ask Sophia what she did in Italy.

Now, hours later, Ronnie was awake when Sophia made her rounds. She opened the door and pointed her small lit flashlight at his chest to make sure he was breathing. Old habits die hard, she thought.

"Hey, Sophia."

"Oh, Hi, Ronnie. I didn't mean to wake you. Just wanted to make sure you were alright. Can I get you anything?"

"No, I'm fine. Do you feel like talking?" he asked.

"Sure." Sophia sat down in the chair next to his bed after she turned on the bathroom light so it wasn't too bright in the room.

"You know what you said earlier tonight about my family?"

Sophia thought she did not even come close to saying what she wanted to say. This was the son of the man who outlawed gay marriage, the loving union Terri and Leslie built, and Sura and Liz, and so many others.

"You mean about not having the experiences yet to look at things in different ways?"

"Yeah, that's what I mean. It got me thinking. I like this girl in one of my classes last semester."

"What's her name, Ronnie?"

"Alessandra."

"That's pretty."

"Yeah. She is and smart too. She's from Peru. Here on scholarship."

"That's real nice. So, what's the problem, Ronnie?"

"Too dark. Not American."

"For you or your parents?"

"Does it matter?" Ronnie said.

JUNE 9, 2021 4:00 A.M.
National Health Center, Respiratory Unit, Staff Lounge

Sophia felt tired. Even though she was usually awake at this time she usually had sleep, albeit broken, in the hours leading up to this one.

She poured a cup of coffee and sipped. She did not need any cream.

"Good coffee," she said to Charlie who just entered the room.

"Ain't no sense in drinking a shitty cup," he said.

"Is it finally time for a wee break?" Jack said closing the door behind him.

"I'm just glad to get them with y'all FNGs here," Charlie said.

"What's an FNG?" Jack asked.

Sophia jumped in. "Fuck'n New Guy or Gal, in my case."

"Or FOG in my case now, Sophia," Charlie smiled.

Jack sat down and asked Charlie what he knew about the Smiths. Charlie explained Sam had been ventilated most of the time he took care of him, and his wife spoke more to the female nurses, especially Tina.

Jack wanted to know if Charlie knew anything about their relationship with Bart Sawyer who was being discharged tomorrow.

"I know they know each other from Birmingham, way down in Alabama. Mrs. Smith stopped in to see Sawyer when her husband was still alive, before she became one of the patients," Charlie said.

"Do you think Smith and Sawyer worked together?" Jack asked.

"I don't know. I don't like a lot of talking. That's why I try and stay in the ICU."

"Right then, Charlie. I'm just trying to understand is all. Mrs. Smith asked me if Bart was still sick. I told her he was going home in the morn. Then she got to wondering if Bart's pig was sick like Sam's. I couldn't sort all that out.

"And I sure as hell couldn't ask Bart Sawyer himself about any of it. He hasn't said much at all tonight except, 'You sure do talks funny like all dem people we have everywhere we look. Least your skin ain't too dark.'"

"Yeah, there are some nasty racists in this bunch. You should hear Johnson when he gets going. Well, that's when he could still talk," Charlie said.

"I don't take any offense me self, but it sure got me thinking how I haven't seen hatred like that in a man's eye since me old misty past back home," Jack said.

"Hey, where's that, Jack?" Sophia asked as she poured a second cup of coffee. "You never did say exactly where you're from in Ireland."

"It's a story for the ages, to be sure, love."

Bloody Sunday, 1972
Londonderry, Northern Ireland

Not many Catholics died on January 30 in the Bogside, their very own neighborhood in the British, Protestant-ruled north except for Patrick Doherty, Jack's father. Patrick's chest was the unlucky recipient of the bullet from the bodachs, that's what the Irish Catholics called the Brits, who had fired their guns willy-nilly on this day in defense of the sounds of their own bullets ricocheting off the building walls.

Jack, the oldest son, stood with his father in protest, earlier in the day, against the soldiers barricading them in the Bogside so the Catholics could not march to the city center demanding access to jobs only given to Protestants. Without these jobs, the Bogside denizens could not make the money they needed to pay their taxes and get some political representation locally and nationally.

When Patrick fell to the ground, Jack started throwing rocks at the soldiers who in turn took care of Jack with the force of their sticks. An hour later, Jack came to, but only to find his father lying in a pool of blood.

Mary Doherty's response to Jack's news, when he ran home to make sure the rest of the family was safe before going back out to tend to the fallen Catholics, might have made anyone else think she did not care too much about Patrick.

"We're mov'n on then, as fast as we can, in the morn, to Liverpool. Me sister did it few years back when all these Troubles began," she announced without a tear in her eye or a crack in her voice.

Mary Doherty remained strong for her three sons and four daughters by only grieving at night when she was alone as she could be in a closet in her sister's home. But Jack could hear her sobs and curses at God for taking her Patrick.

Jack longed for Londonderry after they reached Liverpool. They moved into the two-bedroom home of Mary's sister on Hanover Street near the Mersey River. Only this block was safe for the Irish. At least back home, Jack had a whole neighborhood and school filled with other Irish Catholics.

The teachers at their new school called all of the Doherty boys "Paddy" and the girls "Bridget." The English boys hurled "dirty Mick" epithets at Jack along with their fists when they followed him home. After a while they stopped, only because Jack never backed down.

JUNE 9, 2021, 4:15 A.M.
National Health Center, Respiratory Unit, Staff Lounge

"So, Jack, how'd you become a nurse?" Sophia asked.

"Me Mum always told me to stick it out in school. University was paid for if you got your A levels, sort of like completing your first year of college here. I wanted to do a bit more than sitting in a classroom for years listening to old farts tell me about the world.

"The nursing schools were opening up more to men then. I knew it would suit me just fine ever since I helped out old doc patch up the wounded on Bloody Sunday in the Bogside."

"Damn straight, Jack. I would've been on the streets myself if I hadn't taken my medic training from Nam into Nashville's hospital diploma program. They took in me and two other guys in '72," Charlie said.

"To be sure, Charlie. I could've taken a dangerous path me self. But I ended up at St. Bart's nursing school in London. When I graduated in 1978, I swore I'd never live under British rule ever again"

"You picked the right country here, Jack," Charlie said. "Well, at least then."

"To be sure. I was hired at Village Community in New York City when I graduated and by 1980 I had me green card. By 1984 I was a full-fledged American citizen and AIDS nurse."

"Better you than me, buddy," Charlie said and shot out of the room.

Jack was walking with Reba Smith from the bathroom to her bed making sure she did not trip on the long oxygen tubing in her nostrils connected to the wall. She was still short of breath when she was not resting, and she needed to go to the bathroom every hour or so due to the diarrhea.

"Thank you, sweetie. You're very kind," she said to Jack.

"No worries, love. You just get yourself back in the bed now and I'll set you up for your bath. Our aide, Cheryl, will be in to help you soon enough," Jack said.

Reba Smith asked Jack if he could ask Bart Sawyer to stop in and see her before he went home today. "I likes to talk with someone who knew my Sam." Then she cried.

"That will be a bit of comfort for you. There's a good amount of hurt in there right now," Jack placed his hand over his heart. "It must feel like a knife. That'll take some time to not feel so sharp, Mrs. Smith."

"That Bart is, I means was, a good friend to my Sam. Theys did their charity work together," Reba said.

"Is that what the pigs were for, Mrs. Smith?"

Reba explained they got pigs for the blind children's Christmas dinner every year and for their own. "But that one we had this past Christmas was real sick. It got me thinking maybe that's what got my Sam so sick."

"What happened to the pig then, Mrs. Smith?"

She explained Sam killed the pig when she drove all the way to Birmingham for a good Christmas ham. Then Jack asked her how she knew the pig was so ill.

"It just stood there, out in the pen, didn't move at all. And it sure looked a little purple. I thought I could ask Bart if the pig he got was that sick."

"You're thinking his might not have been because he's going home?"

"I'm just thinking. Trying to figure it all out," Mrs. Smith said still trying to catch her breath.

JUNE 9, 2021, 6:45 A.M.
National Health Center, Respiratory Unit

Sophia made sure Betty Ann Williams was comfortable sitting up in her bedside chair with a pillow behind her lower back, a warm blanket draped over her legs propped up on a small stool while Sophia totaled up her intake and output of fluids for the shift. Her calculations proved the patient was taking in far more than what she was putting out, indicating her kidney function was worsening.

"Have a good day, Mrs. Williams."

"Please call me Betty Ann, Nurse."

"Only if you call me Sophia."

As Sophia opened the bedroom door to the anteroom, a handsome middle-aged man was standing there.

"Howdy, Nurse. I understand my little sweetheart's in here. I've been driving all night to see her. I'm Burt Williams."

"Well, hello, Mr. Williams. I'm your wife's nurse, Sophia."

"She said you was a looker. Middle Eastern or something like that."

Sophia just smiled. There was no sense in correcting him now.

Sophia went to Ronnie Lynch's room next. She knew the transporter would be coming up to the unit any minute now to take him to dialysis. "Ronnie, you good in there?" she raised her voice so he could hear her behind the closed bathroom door.

His face was clean and his hair was wet and combed back

when he opened the door. "I'm just fine. Thank you for everything, Sophia. Will you be on tonight?"

"Sure will be. See you around eightish, right after report."

The Black transporter knocked on the door and opened it. "Mr. Lynch, Good morning. Your chariot awaits you."

Sophia noticed Ronnie did not say hello or even smile at the transporter as he walked to the wheelchair in the hallway.

"Thank you so much, Alex," Sophia said after she read his name tag. Then she touched Alex's shoulder and said, "Have a good one."

The transporter smiled and said, "Thank you, Nurse. You do the same."

Sophia was walking towards the staff lounge. It was almost time to give report now. She saw Burt Williams walking in the direction of the visitor's kitchen, probably looking for some coffee, she thought, after that long drive, when the transporter wheeled Ronnie Lynch past him heading for the elevator.

Ronnie looked up at Burt and Burt looked down at him. Sophia heard Burt say, "Lord have mercy, Confederate Jack. What on earth are you doing all the way up here? You don't look so good." And she could have sworn Ronnie said, "R. E. Lee?"

JUNE 9, 2021, 7:15 A.M.
National Health Center, Respiratory Unit, Staff Lounge

Sophia had texted Sura during her break because she knew she would be up by then. She asked Sura to meet for some breakfast after her shift was over, and she was looking forward to it now.

Fred Johnson was on duty today for the first time and he was a little nervous about how he was going to handle these patients. Jack assured him that being Mid-Western, white, and lacking a foreign accent would carry him far with this lot, plus Bart Sawyer was going home.

Jack explained Reba Smith was preoccupied with her sadness over her husband's death and James Wilson slept most of the night.

"When I did talk with him for a wee minute this morn he asked me where I was from and I told him Northern Ireland. Then he asked me how long I had been here, and I told him I became an American citizen back in the '80s.

'Oh, the right way,' he said. 'None of that illegal shit. And you at least speak English I can understand.'"

"Can't wait," Fred said.

"Just don't share too much about yourself, Fred, if you know what I mean," Jack winked.

"No worries there."

Jack finished his report with all of the clinical details on his patients, and then Sophia began report the way Jack ended. She described Betty Ann Williams' purple lesions and fluid balance, and Ronnie Lynch's dialysis schedule and ongoing electrolyte imbalances.

Then she turned to the more personal information she learned about Ronnie.

Thomas said, "That's peculiar, Sophia, I would not have thought he had any interest in girls."

"Well, he's the one who brought up this girl in his class. But I know what you mean, Thom, after what I just saw in the hallway."

"What was that, then?" Jack asked.

"Ronnie was passing Mr. Williams, who just arrived from Georgia, on his way to dialysis, and they exchanged words," Sophia said.

"They know each other?" Thom asked.

"You're bloody kidding me," Jack said.

"How in the world could they?" Thom said. "The Vice President of the Unites States' son and what does Mr. Williams do, Sophia?"

"His wife said he's a shelfer in Jackson, Georgia. I know it doesn't make sense but I know what I saw, and what I heard," Sophia said.

"What was that exactly?" Thom asked.

"Mr. Williams called Ronnie 'Confederate Jack' and Ronnie referred to him as 'R. E. Lee,'" Sophia said.

"What the fuck is that all about?" Fred asked.

"I do not know, Frederick, but we will find out today," Thom said.

"Frederick? I haven't been called that in a long time. I don't mind though. Let's get busy finding some answers, Thomas."

June 9, 2019, 7:45 A.M.
Crystal Nightingale Hotel Lounge, Crystal City, Va.

Sura was sipping some chamomile tea at a table for two when Sophia rushed in, greeted by the aroma of freshly roasted coffee she knew she could not drink if she wanted to get any sleep today.

"No hurry, sweetie. I'm enjoying this tea," Sura said.

"Thanks for meeting me, Sura. I knew you would be up when I texted you, but I wasn't sure if you would be up for a bite."

"Usually I sleep for a few hours during the night, but I'm always awake at 4 o'clock. Then I'm able to go back to sleep around nine for a few more hours, since I've been retired anyway."

"I'm always up at four, too, Sura. And then I can't go back to sleep when I have to be at work by nine."

"For your counseling in Florence?"

"Yes. It's weird though, isn't it, Sura? It's like we're still programmed to be the night watchwomen for the dying."

"They did always seem to go in that hour, didn't they?"

"Always," Sophia said.

"How was your first night back on duty?"

"It was good to take care of patients again. They're pretty sick too, physically and emotionally, especially the young one."

"The VIP?" Sura asked.

"Yes."

"Did you have any memories?"

"Reynaldo from Brazil. The female patient I took care of had those purple lesions on her abdomen."

"I remember Reynaldo's face. That poor young man."

"Hey, Sura, what have you and Liz been up to?"

"And Cal, and Linda. We've been sightseeing. Cal never really explored all of the D.C. museums, even though she's been here a few times with Teddy. But that's always a family visit," she said.

Sura told Sophia she returned to *The Holocaust Museum* alone yesterday.

"So, are you related to that docent, Mr. Lichtenstein?"

"Fairly, to say the least," Sura said.

Lenny Lichtenstein was Sura Weber's first cousin, her mother's brother, Harvey's, first born. Sura found out yesterday that her mother never told her about her brother's family being captured during Kristallnacht and taken to Dachau.

Lenny told Sura all about their grandparents. He said, "I used to sneak over to Opa and Oma's barracks in the early morning hours. I was only eight when we arrived. The three of us in the smallest wooden frame stuffed with straw the little mice shared with us, too."

Sura said to Sophia, "I told him it must have been wonderful just to be with them."

Then Lenny told Sura about how they died, how they were shot during the march to Tegernsee. They were too weak to walk. "That's when the Nazis made those of us who were left in Dachau march for days, right before the liberation. They did not want us to be free, ever," he told Sura.

Lenny said his own mother was very sick. "She probably had cancer when I think about it now. She vomited every time she ate," he told Sura. "They shot her too when she collapsed on the road."

Sura then told Sophia Lenny and his father made it to Switzerland after the war. Lenny became a History professor and that's when he met his wife, an American graduate student, where he taught at the university.

They married and settled here in Baltimore where they raised their three children.

"I hugged him for a long time, Sophia. It felt good to have family alive in this world. Then he led me to the artifacts room."

Sura described the plate. It was broken but the intact side was decorated with a pink stemmed rose. Sura told Lenny it looked like the plate Oma used to serve her pretzels on. He agreed.

Lenny said it was almost impossible to confirm if it was Oma's plate, but the museum had verified its origin as Dusseldorf. Sura told Lenny she would like them to stay in touch, and he invited her and her spouse to meet his wife, Bonita, last evening.

"She welcomed me like a sister, Sophia. She prepared pretzels that tasted just like Oma's It turns out Lenny had memorized Oma's recipe. She recited it every night in the camp like a tale never to be forgotten."

"That is so wonderful, Sura," Sophia said as their poached eggs over spinach and brioche arrived.

"It is, but after we returned to the hotel last night I could not sleep a wink. It felt like Hans Gruber was sitting in the chair next to my side of the bed, staring at me with those steely blue eyes."

"You mean that patient of ours like in 1992 or '93? The Nazi?"

"Yes. Sophia. The Nazi."

Sura always felt cold inside when she thought about Hans. She figured it was because she remembered him in the context of that winter they took care of him, but that winter was rather temperate. Last night, though, she discovered the deep chill stemmed from what she had kept buried inside for so many years.

Hans was not one of their typical patients. He was not a drug user. He denied any blood transfusions before 1985. He did not indicate he ever engaged in unsafe sex with other men or women. He had no partner, no children, only a sister, Freida, who was even more reticent than him.

It was as if Hans Gruber popped into existence the day he visited the ER at The Upper East Side Medical Center with abdominal pain and vomiting. A 68-year-old white male with a thick German accent who said he had lived in the "Americas" for most of his life now.

The doctors could not find any old medical records. They would have never even thought to test Hans for HIV except for the lymphoma, they found in his abdominal cavity during the exploratory surgery, that came back as Burkitt's, a type usually only seen in AIDS patients.

Sura cared for Hans a lot because of the chemotherapy he

needed. Plus, she knew he was German and he often spoke to her in their native tongue. But Sura suspected he also knew she was Jewish, even though she never mentioned or indicated it in anyway.

"Remind me why you thought he knew," Sophia said.

"I never did tell you, Sophia, because I had forgotten all of this. Hans never let me touch him without gloves. He always said it was for my protection. I assured him it was safe for me.

"One night when our aide, Celia, helped Hans change his gown when I was giving him his chemo, she was not wearing gloves. She even rubbed some lotion on his back. He did not say a word."

Hans' cancer just kept getting worse and the HIV crossed into his brain causing, what appeared to be to the nurses, some pretty awful dementia before he died.

Sophia said, "I remember how terrified he was. All of us saw that. We would wrap him in blankets and hold him tightly to calm him down. He kept repeating, 'The things I've done. The things I've done' with a monstrous look in his eyes."

"Yes. I did hear him say that too, Sophia. But he said a little more than that to me during his last night on this earth."

"I don't remember you telling me about that Sura. You know all of us thought he was a Nazi. He was the right age, German, we knew so little about him, and those words he repeated over and over again every time he got scared."

"That was what I remembered last night, Sophia. The reason I *knew* he was a Nazi."

When Sura checked in on Hans around 1:00 A.M. he was in the bathroom. She came back within the hour and he was still in there. She asked him if he was alright and she could hear him say "Ja" behind the door. But she kept hearing a sound, like the sweeping of a brush on the tiled floor.

Sura did not ask for permission to open the door. She saw

Hans holding a broom, probably left behind by a housekeeper, like a shovel he kept scraping on the floor and lifting up.

"Like he was digging?" Sophia asked.

"Yes, like he was trying to make a hole but knew on some level that he was not getting anywhere. He looked at me and shouted, 'You, Jüden. Get back in there!' and pointed to the floor."

"My God, Sura. How horrific. What did you do then? I mean you must have known he was purely out of his mind."

"Thank goodness Tom was on with me that night because Han's pajama bottoms were saturated with blood in the back all the way down his legs. I did not notice until we got him back into bed.

"He never stopped bleeding. We packed his rectum with surgical pads."

"I remember the bleeding. You told me about that the next night when I was on duty with you."

"I wish I would have never remembered any of it," Sura said as she set her fork on her plate without touching her eggs.

JUNE 9, 2021, 11:30 A.M.
National Health Center, Respiratory Unit

James Wilson had just returned from dialysis and Fred was in his room making sure the correct intravenous fluids were hanging after reading the new orders from the nephrologist.

Fred also signed out some Lomotil for Mr. Wilson because the dialysis nurse had called about an hour and one half ago reporting, really complaining, about the diarrhea the patient had in the reclining chair during his treatment.

"Hi there, Mr. Wilson. We only had a minute to meet each other before you left earlier."

"It's Fred, isn't it?" Mr. Wilson asked.

"Yes, sir. How are you feeling?"

"A little dizzy."

"Dialysis can do that to you. Let me check your blood pressure."

It was low: 80/40. Fred laid the patient flat and made the head of the bed a little lower than the feet. A few minutes later, Fred rechecked the blood pressure: 100/60.

"Much better, Mr. Wilson," Fred said while slowly elevating the head of the bed.

"Thank you. That's right kind of you, Fred. Now tell me, where you from?"

"Outside of Chicago. That's where I grew up. How about you, Mr. Wilson?"

"Rabun County. Clayton. Outside of Atlanta."

"I've always wanted to visit. What kind of work do you do down there?"

"Me and the Mrs., Emmy Lou, have a little café, Jimmy's. Serve breakfast and dinner every day, except Sundays. We're closed in the afternoons."

"What kind of food?"

"Collards, sweet potatoes, chicken, of course, and the best biscuits you'll find until you reach the Alabama line. Emmy Lou's secret family recipe."

"That sounds real nice, Mr. Wilson."

"The only thing now is that new damn dinner theater is practically running us out of business."

James Wilson explained Alvin in Wonderland popped up like a bad weed just one mile outside of Clayton proper in the middle of nowhere, but that did not stop people coming from miles around.

What Mr. Wilson did not know was that these dinner theatres were a subsidiary of President Rumpel's main restaurant chain, Big Al's. The new restaurants catered to regional cuisines. So this one in Rabun county served everything Jimmy's did, plus cocktails.

Mr. Wilson told Fred what he did know. "Tell you what, it's bad enough that damn place is stealing my customers, now there's a whole bunch of slimy I don't know whats working there. And not just one kind.

"Only reason I know that is ever since Wonderland opened up them Mexican criminals have been puttin' up their own food stands, side of the road with beans and tacos smelling up the air with their foulness on Route 76. They're like cockaroaches, I tell you.

"And then Salvadorads work there, too, and do their own popups when they ain't at that theater. And it's even worse with their tortillas and that yuk stuff."

"I believe you mean yucca, Mr. Wilson. It's a vegetable," Fred interrupted.

"Never mind that. That theater's been hiring all them types and ain't one of them legal."

Fred kept a tight lid on his anger as he listened to Mr. Wilson by thinking about home back in the Castro and delicious Mexican dinners with his husband, Li, in the Mission.

"So, Mr. Wilson, have you ever thought about opening your own place, like in Atlanta. It sounds like what you and your wife make is real authentic. You could attract people in the big city in search of some real down-home cooking."

"I won't lie, Fred. I've thought about it. It costs too much for Emmy Lou and me to live there. My daughter, Sue Ellen, moved there a few years ago. Doesn't come home much at all. She has a job that pays her a whole lot of money, though, designing clothes for them damn rappers."

"Do you get to see her?" Fred kept the focus on the patient's daughter.

"Sure do, for a minute or two when I go there to plan my charity work."

"What kind of work do you do?" Fred asked without revealing his skepticism about this man having a charitable bone in his body.

"We help out them blind children. We meet at a place for all the good 'ol boys, if you know what I mean," Mr. Wilson winked.

"Let me know where it is sometime. It's nice to have somewhere to go when you visit a new city. Like I said, I've been meaning to get there," Fred said.

"Just tell them at JD's on Route 85 before you reach downtown that I sent you. Best damn liquor to wet your lips there."

"Sure will, Mr. Wilson. You get some rest now," Fred said and shut his door behind him. "Fuck'n shit. What an asshole," he whispered under his breath while he removed his gown and then washed his hands in the anteroom.

JUNE 9, 2021, 6:15 P.M.
National Health Center, Respiratory Unit

Ronnie Lynch's dialysis days were starting to drain him so much, he just stayed in bed after returning to his room.

Yesterday morning, Dr. Brugge shared his concern with the nurses about how Ronnie was headed towards a kidney transplant if the cause of his disease was not found soon. And the purple lesions were not going anywhere except down Ronnie's swollen legs.

Thomas Bechtel could see, during this last round before evening report, that the young man was not feeling well. "You've had a difficult time here, Ronnie. I'm sure you were looking forward to some enjoyment this summer."

"Well, I would be in Greece now with my parents. So, yes, it would have been some enjoyment, not a lot, but it sure would beat this."

"Do you have any pain right now, Ronnie?"

"Some in my legs. They are so big now. But mainly in my heart."

"Point to it, if you will," Thomas wanted to make sure the pain was not cardiac in nature.

"I can't. It's so deep inside," he started crying.

"You can share with me, if you like, Ronnie."

Ronnie dropped the JD's napkin he was clutching in his hand onto the bed. "He said I could call him anytime, but when I did a few minutes ago he said he couldn't talk because he was on the road."

"It's hard, Ronnie. The first one always is. Believe me, I know," Thomas said after picking up the napkin.

"But I really thought he would come and see me," Ronnie said.

"From down in Georgia?" Thomas asked reading the address on the napkin.

"No, Thom, from down the hallway. I saw him on my way to dialysis this morning."

"You rest up now, Ronnie. Tomorrow is a new day and a dialysis-free one," Thomas said and covered him with a blanket.

He shut the door, washed his hands, and ran to the break-room to call Ashley Smith.

June 10, 2021, 6:58 A.M.
National Health Center, Respiratory Unit, Staff Lounge

"I'm nervous, shug. I ain't gonna lie," Cal said to Sophia while adding four packets of sugar to her coffee cup.

"You shouldn't be, Cal. You're still nursing."

"I detest facing such ugliness, though. That Dan Napolina, by the way, Sophia, he's a real nice one and a cutie, told me when I saw him yesterday in our hotel how nasty that Mr. Johnson and some of the others are."

"Well, Cal, Mr. Johnson is not a problem now on the ventilator. But you're going to do just fine. You always do. Did. Plus, you get to work your first shift with Fred. It'll be just like home in San Francisco," Sophia said.

"Hey everyone," Fred said as he came in the room. He explained to Cal that the float nurse from ICU will take care of Johnson and he will take care of James Wilson again and Ronnie Lynch. "That leaves the two ladies for you, Cali girl."

"Just like home, like you said, Sophia. Fred never tires of bossing me around,' Cal said smiling.

Bridgette had come in a few minutes ago, ready to end the long night shift.

"Reba Smith is harmless enough, Cal. More concerned right now about her daughter travelling up here from Birmingham than about her own grief."

"Oh, that's right. The poor thing. Her husband just died this past Saturday, didn't he, the day we all learned about this whole thing. It feels like it's been weeks, and this is only my first shift,' Cal said.

Bridgette first reported the details about Reba Smith's antibiotic schedule, her IV site and the type of fluids infusing, the shift total of her fluids in and out, the frequency of her diarrhea finally starting to slow down, and her appetite. "She ate some green beans and potatoes last evening for dinner. Still not hungry for meat." And then Bridgette told Cal everything they knew so far, thanks to Jack's conversations the night before this one.

"Maybe that's why her husband died. Maybe he did get

something from that sick pig. I don't know how, but it's possible," Cal replied.

Sophia gave Cal report on Betty Ann Williams, beginning with her worsening kidney function and the initiation of renal dose Dopamine ordered by Dr. Brugge last night to increase blood flow to her kidneys and hopefully delay the need for dialysis.

Cal started to think about the monitoring required with this intravenous medication and the hourly urine measurements. "She has a Foley catheter in, right, Sophia?"

Sophia nodded and said, "Just like riding a bike, Cal. First time, I got right into the bladder."

Cal wrote down the hourly routine for this patient: checking urine output, blood pressure, pulse, respiratory rate, oxygen saturation level, skin color, IV site.

"How are her veins, Sophia?" Cal remembered if the Dopamine drip infused into the patient's tissue instead of the vein, it could cause necrosis.

"Thank God they placed a central line yesterday, one of those dialysis catheters," Sophia said.

Lastly, she told Cal about the size and location of Mrs. Williams' purple lesions.

"Do we know what they are yet?" Cal asked.

"No one knows," Sophia said

"The disease must be affecting the blood vessels underneath the skin to cause that color," Cal said.

"Good point," Sophia said. "But what we do know is Betty Ann Williams' husband, Burt, does the same kind of charity work for albino children like the rest of these guys."

"Why albinos?" Cal asked.

"I don't know. But an even more interesting piece in this whole unsolved puzzle is Mrs. Williams' husband knows Ronnie Lynch," Sophia said.

"The Vice President's son? Whooee! How do you know?" Cal said.

"I saw and heard the two of them exchange words yesterday morning. Burt Williams drove up here from Georgia to see his wife and he and Ronnie saw each other in the hallway when Ronnie was on his way to dialysis. They called each other nicknames, like Civil War era ones," Sophia explained.

"Kinky, girl. Like what?" Cal asked.

"Williams called Ronnie 'Confederate Jack' and Ronnie called him 'R. E. Lee.'"

"Lordy be!" Cal said.

Fred now interjected. "And Thomas has been taking care of Ronnie who he said was in tears last evening when he tried to call this R. E. Lee who could not talk because he was on his way back to Georgia."

Sophia jumped in. "That's right. And Thomas said R.E. Lee's name and number were on a JD's napkin Ronnie dropped on his bed."

"Unreal! Where is this JD's again?" Cal asked.

"Atlanta. Just like Gerald and Ashley mentioned last Saturday night," Fred said.

"Someone needs to check out that place," Cal commented.

"Thomas and I are one ahead of you, Cali. Road trip tomorrow. We're both off," Fred said.

"Oooh, I wish I could go along. I know some fine bars down there," Cal said.

"It doesn't sound like this bar is one of them," Fred said.

"Yeah, from what I've heard, these men do not seem too 'out' at all. Just as well, I'd like to see what I can find out right here about the husbands of these ladies, the dead one and the Georgian," Cal said.

"You were always the best at drawing out information,

Cal," Sophia said. "Remember when you got that frail young woman to talk, the one we took care of in Room 5 in 1990 or '91? Must have been 1991 because that's when you joined us."

Sophia told all of the nurses in the room how no one could get this woman to open up about why her mouth always bled in the evenings after dinner. "Do you remember her name, Cal?"

"Val. Valentina. She was one terrified, or shall I say terrorized, little thing," Cal remarked.

"She sure was. I even talked to her in Spanish. She would give excuses like the food was too 'caliente' or áspero, you know hot or rough, and that's why she bled. But Cal here got her to say her husband shoved the fork into her mouth over and over again at dinner time every night behind the curtain he drew around her bed," Sophia said.

Cal told all of them. "Sophia is so right. Val told me, I kid you not, what that man said to her as he did it, 'Eat bitch, eat. If you get any thinner, they'll blame me for your AIDS."

"Wow," Bridgette said, "What a fuck'n bastard."

"Oh, he was, honey. I made sure after that the day shift aide or our Tom on nights fed Valentina dinner before her husband got off work. He was real mad when he came in every night after that.

"I used to smile and say, 'Mr. Perez we took care of your wife. No worries there, sweetie.' And back then I wasn't half the alluring woman I am today!" she snapped her fingers up high in the air.

"You were always all that, Cal, and so much more," Sophia said.

Cal walked over to Sophia and gave her a big hug.

June 10, 2021, 12:00 P.M.
National Health Center, Respiratory Unit

Cal had no choice but to spend most of her morning with Betty Ann Williams. It took Cal almost a half an hour to perform the required hourly checks associated with her Dopamine drip.

"Nurse Moore, you've been a God-send today. I don't know what I'd do without you and the exotic one on nights. I never thought, dear, that you dark folks could have ever helped me like this."

"Please call me Cal, Mrs. Williams. You know it's funny," Cal said with a big smile on her face, "I never thought I would like to care for someone so white."

"Who on earth do you usually take care of, Cal?"

"People of all colors, gay people, straight people, and plenty of other stripes too."

"My heavens, Cal, where are you from? I thought you were a right proper Southern gal."

"Born and bred in Mississippi, Ma'am, but my heart's always in San Francisco."

"Where they have no rules about proper conduct," Mrs. Williams said.

"Well, let's see. No one judges you for who you are there. People try and respect differences. That's perdy proper ain't it, Mrs. Williams?"

"I suppose it all depends on how you look at things, doesn't it?"

"'Deed it does, Mrs. Williams. It's all in the way you approach people."

The patient then began to tell Cal about her son, Joel, a lawyer in Washington, D.C. who moved there after law school.

"You must be real proud," Cal said.

"I sure am. Burt, my husband, not so much. Joel's a liberal. He works for the CLO."

"A sin, indeed!" Cal said.

The patient laughed out loud. Cal saw her reach for her abdomen.

"How bad is that pain, Mrs. Williams?"

"Not too terrible."

"May I take a look?"

The patient said yes. Cal examined her abdomen. The lesions now were starting to look like a wave of irregularly shaped lilies floating ashore around her back.

Stephen on the AIDS Unit at Upper East Side Medical from 1992 appeared in the bed now. Cal closed the door on that memory. She needed to stay focused on Mrs. Williams.

"I can get you some hydrocodone tablets, or something stronger for your pain, Mrs. Williams. Give me a number from one to ten, one is minor and ten is the worse pain you ever had, not including childbirth, which is always a fifteen."

The patient started to laugh again and Cal said, "My apologies. Now take some slow, deep breaths."

"It's about a four, Cal."

"I'll be right back with some hydrocodone."

"You are very kind, dear," Mrs. Williams said.

Cal returned within ten minutes with a fresh pitcher of water. She poured the patient some water and handed her two pills in a medication cup. "If this doesn't work within the hour, I'll get the doc to order something stronger."

"Thank you so much, Cal. It's funny how you brought up judgement, judging people a little whiles ago. I've been plenty guilty of it with my own Burt."

"Your husband?"

"'Deed I have. I used to get so upset when he came back home from his overnight visits to Atlanta for his charity work."

"You miss him when he's gone, of course."

"Well, yes, I do. But it's his closeness with his friends that always bothers me."

"Men, Mrs. Williams, sometimes need a little more than what we can give them as wives," Cal said.

"I just can't understand why he needs that kind of inter-course. But I don't judge him no more for it."

"Why do you think he needs that?" Cal asked.

"Who do you think washes the clothing in our house?"

"Oh, I see," Cal said.

"But I prayed and prayed on it, to God Almighty to give me the strength to accept my Burt for needing so much more. And the Lord hasn't failed me yet."

"You rest now, Mrs. Williams. Let those pain pills do their magic," Cal said and walked out of her room into the anteroom to de-gown and wash her hands.

"I do declare," Cal said under her breath.

JUNE 10, 2021, 5:00 P.M.
National Health Center, Respiratory Unit

"Miss Reba, I truly apologize for neglecting you today," Cal said as she rushed back into Mrs. Smith's room to make sure the 4:00 P.M. antibiotic finished infusing.

"You take real good care of me today, Nurse Cal. And thank the good Lord I had some time to visit with my daughter."

"Well then, where's she now? She came all that way to see you."

"I believe I upset my Mary Joe."

"Why I don't believe it, Mrs. Smith. She seemed right pleased to see you when she arrived this morning."

"Now I knows you my nurse but I never confided in no dark person before."

"Miss Reba, try not to remind me why I never have any desire to go back home to Mississippi."

"Forgive my manners, Nurse Cal. I never used to talk that way in public. Used to always scold my Sam when he did."

"I can see how upset you are, Mrs. Smith. I thought you might like to share."

"I feel right comfortable with you, Nurse Cal. I know I shouldn't feel that way with no nig ...I mean, Black person, but I do."

Reba Smith told Cal all about the conversation she had with her daughter before Mary Joe turned right back around after a fourteen-hour car drive that began last night at 6:30 P.M.

Mary Joe knew how sick her father was but she had no desire to visit him here in Virginia before he died. She only talked to him when she absolutely needed to, ever since she married Luther a few years ago and Sam Smith refused to attend their wedding.

"Now, Pa, people in my generation don't have no problem with people who ain't white and you shouldn't know how neither. Luther's a good man, a teacher and I loves him," Mary Joe said to her father in the Smiths' kitchen the night before her marriage.

"I don't care if he's as rich as President Rumpel, my daughter has disgraced our family going and marrying one of dem people," Sam said.

Mary Joe still saw her mother. Reba Smith even visited them in their home. She always told her daughter, "Mary Joe, I love to hear your Luther talk. He talks just like a white man from the north. Sounds real smart."

And Mary Joe would say, "He talks like that Mama cause

he is real smart. Went to college all the ways up there in Connecticut."

"Well, my Mary Joe's pretty smart too," Reba would tell her. "You just don't sound that way on account of me and your Pa."

"Luther tells me I'm smart all the time. I'm just so glad I got that job as the principal's secretary at Luther's school. That's how we met, you know. And now I get to take classes for free at the university," she had told her mother.

It was what Mary Joe had told her mother this morning in her hospital room that led to her departure. Right before Christmas, on December 20, she had driven over to her parents' house to see if Reba wanted to go with her to the big market in Birmingham. She knew the Christmas pig her father brought home from North Carolina at Halloween was too ill to eat, so her mother had told her.

Mary Joe knew when she arrived she should have called ahead because no one was in the house when she entered. She walked out the kitchen door to the barn. Reba's car was gone but there were a few pickup trucks parked in front of the closed barn door.

Mary Joe moved one of the crates her father used for picking vegetables over to the light shining through the small barn window. She told her mother this morning that she never mentioned what she saw that day because she was still trying to make sense of it all.

"Pa and some other men killed that little pig in the barn."

"I know that, Mary Joe. Your Pa said he was taking care of the poor little thing when I went to the market," Reba said to her daughter.

"Yeah but Ma, Pa led those men in saying they had to keep the white race alive. And they all had them hoods on. Then one of them took an axe to that pig's head and they all removed their hoods. They started placing blood crosses on their foreheads. I stepped down when they did that. I couldn't take no more."

Reba Smith told Cal now, "I called my daughter a liar, said she just wants to hurt her Dadddy's memory cause he never could accept her marriage."

"Lordy, Mrs. Smith," Cal said.

"That's right, Nurse Cal. I don't know if she's madder at me for call'n her husband that word or her a liar. But before she left she told me, 'Ma, I only told you this now in case that pig's the reason Pa got sick and died. Might be why you're sick too.'

"Then she told me, Nurse Cal, she never wants to speak to me again." Reba started crying so hard then. "I needs her, Nurse. I loves her so. I even love Luther, just never admitted that to no one."

"Let her cool down some, Miss Reba. Call her tomorrow and tell her how sorry you really are."

"I sure will, Nurse Cal. I thank you for listening to my tale of woe."

Cal told the patient he would be back to check in on her before the end of her shift. As Cal washed her hands in the anteroom's sink, she whispered to herself, "I just knew that pig was the culprit."

Ashley Smith had just arrived on the unit to see how Cal's first day on duty went as Cal came out of Mrs. Smith's room.

"Lordy be, Miss Ashley, I've sure learned a good deal today about these women."

"Do you have a minute to chat, Cal?" Ashley asked.

"Not really, Miss Ashley. I forgot how intense the Dopamine drip patients can be. I need to get back to Mrs. Williams now."

Ashley walked with Cal and said, "I should've thought

more about that much earlier. Next shift and thereafter I'll
have a nurse just assigned to Mrs. Williams."

"You're a good one, Miss Ashley. Many supervisors
wouldn't act like that when they see a problem."

Ashley smiled and said, "You're on tomorrow, right?"

Cal nodded and walked into Mrs. Williams' room.

June 11, 2021, 7:15 A.M.
National Health Center, Respiratory Unit, Staff Lounge

Ashley Smith was listening to the night shift's report. Jack and
Bridgette were going off duty and Cal, Dan, and Margarita
were coming on.

Jack told Cal that Reba Smith repeated the story with her
daughter for him. And then both of them gave Ashley the
details about the pig blood ritual Mrs. Smith's daughter
witnessed this past Christmas season.

"Oh my," Ashley responded. "It's starting to make some
sense now, the things we've been hearing all along."

Then Jack reported Mrs. Smith called her daughter late last
night to make sure she made it home alright and to apologize.
"The daughter must've accepted it because then she told her
Mum to tell the doctors and nurses all about the sick pig and
where her father got the little thing in case other people like her
own Da got sick and died."

Ashley asked Jack, "So Did Mrs. Smith tell you the name of
the pig farm?"

"Well, eventually, for sure. She knew the farm was in
North Carolina but could not remember the name. She said it
had the name of an old Looney Tunes character," Jack said.

"What's a Looney Tune?" Ashley asked.

"I've never heard of that either," Margarita said.

"Ya know, it's truly amazing to me," Dan spoke up now, "And no offense to yous two young ladies, but why is it that we have access to everyting now with all this social media. I mean we get to hear and see what so and so ate for dinner and hear about when they took a shit, but Rock Hudson and Greta Garbo and old classic cartoons are like tings from another planet."

Ashley and Margarita burst out laughing. Then Ashley said, "I know my parents are always amazed what I don't know about the past. It's like all our technology enabled us to focus so much on our own lives, we lost sight of the bigger world around us."

Jack resumed his report. He said he had asked Mrs. Smith if she was trying to think of the character, Porky Pig, and she said, "That's it, Jack. Porky's Farm."

Ashley finished taking notes. All of the nurses were leaving the breakroom.

Jack asked Bridgette, "Hey, Bridge, how's about a night cap and a wee bit of breakfast?"

"Are you shitt'n me. I could use one after this shift," she said.

JUNE 11, 2021, 7:50 A.M.
O'Toole's, Crystal City, Va.

This pub provided night shift nurses, lab techs, respiratory therapists, pharmacists, and post-call medical and surgical residents hearty breakfasts, good pints of Guinness and liquor-infused coffees and juices to carry them off to a good day's sleep.

Jack and Bridgette found two quiet seats at the bar. "You know, Bridge, I felt bad for that Mrs. Smith losing her husband and all, and now finding out about that pig ritual bit."

"She must have known something wasn't right about what her husband did, though. I mean she knew he wore a white hood. Who the hell does that for charity work? Was there ever even a charity? And she herself must be one hell of a racist married to that man for all these years."

"I haven't seen so much meself but Cal sure has and the other nurses with any bit of color in them. So, Bridgette, how's that Ronnie been treating you?"

"Oh, just fine because I pass. If he only knew I was gay and married to a Black woman he'd shit. He would also shit with me insisting we're still married after his asshole father got it outlawed.

"He is really very sick, though, Jack. You heard my report. I spent most of the night trying to keep his lungs clear from all the fluid building up in him. He should be in dialysis right now. It'll help but not as much as it should," Bridgette said.

"That Wilson you had last night, seems real challenging, belief-wise that is," she continued.

"To be sure. He's not too, too sick yet, but he's really nasty. I didn't report on half the racist shite he said to me last night. Talked quite a bit about anyone not white and not Southern in that wee little town of his in Georgia, as if the invasion of the fuck'n bloody body snatchers was besetting them all. You know, though, Bridge, who kept paying me mind a visit last night?"

"Let me guess," Bridgette said while taking a big gulp of Guinness, "Cunningham. 1989 or '90."

"I think it was both. It took him that bloody long to die. To this day, Bridge, I swear on my Da's grave, he's the nastiest man I've ever met. I felt bad for him in me heart, but in me mind I couldn't get there in the least," Jack said.

"He was as mean as a junkyard dog."

"I like that one, Bridge."

Jack and Bridgette talked about how Ronald Cunningham was found face down on the corner of Bleeker and 6th Avenue, Thanksgiving night, 1989. The cop saw he was still breathing so he brought him into the ER at Village Community Center.

Mr. Cunningham was drunk and looked like he had not eaten for months, weighing only 90 pounds and standing, when he could, at 5 feet and 11 inches. He had one hell of a cough and felt as hot as a ready tea kettle. That's how Jack remembered it when he admitted the patient on the AIDS Ward up on the seventh floor after the doctor tested his blood for HIV antibodies, the only way to check then, and his sputum for tuberculosis.

Ronald Cunningham arrived on Jack's floor coughing and cursing through the mask, when he kept it on. "You rotten motherfuckers. You white bastard," he called Jack.

"Oh, yeah. I remember how much he hated white people, Jack," Bridgette said.

"He hated everyone, really, didn't he, then," Jack said as their plates of runny eggs, blood pudding, kidney beans, and sourdough toast were set in front of them by the bartender.

"That first night he came up to our ward, I got him in isolation as soon as I could. Lord knows how many of us became too familiar with his TB, the bacteria just orbiting around us every time he removed his mask."

"He always tried to spit in your face or throw a bloody tissue at you while telling us we all deserved AIDS like him," Bridgette said in between some bites.

It took months for his TB to become inactive. Mr. Cunningham would pack the INH and Rifampin pills in his cheek pretending to swallow them, and then spit them out after the nurses left his room.

"Do you remember, Bridge, when he escaped that one

night in search of some heroin, his wee 'pick me up' as he liked to call it."

"Sure do. That time he was found face down on 2nd and Avenue B about a month later," Bridgette said.

When Ronald Cunningham came back into Village Community he weighed 80 pounds., and had *PCP* pneumonia. It took months for his pneumonia to resolve and by then his diarrhea from *Cryptococcus*, the nastiest of bugs, began.

"I never saw anyone shit like that before," Bridgette said as she took another sip of Guinness and Jack began his second pint. "He never got off of his bedside commode."

"Not long after that then, Bridge, he couldn't get out of his bed. That poor lad was awfully weak."

"But still mean as hell. And he just kept getting thinner. I never saw anyone that thin, not out of the grave anyway," Bridgette said.

"The last time we weighed him during his early morning bath he was 55 pounds and that was with the sheets on the bed scale with him, mind you," Jack said.

"One night on my rounds, Jack, I couldn't see him breathing so I moved my flashlight up to his face. And there were those big brown eyes wide open taking up all of the space in his skull. He looked terrified.

"But that didn't stop him from yelling, 'You fuck'n pale-faced bitch, always making me shit myself and then waking me up," Bridgette said as tears built up in her eyes.

"I don't remember if you were on with me the night he died, Bridge."

She shook her head no.

"He got a big surge of energy, like they do, you know. Cunningham jumped up out of bed and grabbed Mr. Davis' cane nearby, and started swinging at me when I came in the room.

"He shouted, 'You rotten Irish prick. Speak right for a change.'

"I grabbed the end of his stick as he swung it at me and I swung him back into bed because he wouldn't let go of his end. Derek, our aide, as you remember, and me restrained him right quick.

"He never stopped cursing until he finally caught the last train out of this world. That was Christmas morn, 1990. I like to believe, Bridge, the root of his nastiness came from having one lousy life and one lousy virus that made his brain its final resting place.

"Now then, Bridgette, onto a nicer subject before we get our wee rest for the day. Can you tell me how me lost love, your dear, sweet sister, Fiona, is getting on these days? Is she happy?"

"She is, Jack. Her paintings haven't brought her any fame or fortune, but she makes a decent living from selling them out in Arizona."

"Did she marry?"

"Twice. This one is a good one. A High School Arts teacher who loves the hell out of her."

"That's good. She's had two then."

"Not the first husband."

"I meant who love her," Jack said raising his empty pint.

JUNE 11, 2021, 8:15 P.M.
National Health Center, Respiratory Unit, Doctor's Lounge

Ashley Smith had asked Dr. Gerald Brugge yesterday if they could meet to discuss all of the information the nurses had learned about these patients. Ashley made it to most of the shift reports this past week and took lots of notes.

She plopped down in the large, cushiony chair drinking the soy latte machiatto from the lobby café that she knew was too complicated for Gerald's taste so she got him a regular coffee. She was eating some unsalted almonds when he came in.

"Apologies for my lateness," Gerald said.

"Don't be ridiculous, Brugge," she said and handed him the coffee.

"Thank you. I could use it. I needed to speak with the nephrologist. James Wilson's kidneys are worsening in spite of the dialysis. I've managed to save Betty Ann Williams from dialysis with the Dopamine drip, for now anyway. But how are things on your end, Ashley?"

"I'd say pretty darn good. These nurses are something else, what they've discovered in only five days!"

"I thought they could. They have a unique way of relating to challenging patients. Back then it was all the discrimination our AIDS patients experienced, and that happened before they were even diagnosed. And then all of the miserable reactions to their disease from spouses, partners, family, bosses, and unfortunately our own healthcare system, including doctors and nurses.

"These nurses who chose to work with AIDS then gained their patients' trust. They were the only ones who could. They made them feel human and never judged."

"That is so admirable, Gerald."

"It was. And now their challenge has been to not show judgement with these patients who are huge racists and anti-gay experiencing another unknown infectious disease, and to connect with them enough to get them to talk about anything we can use to find the cause of it."

"And talk they did, Gerald, in spite of the nurses belonging to these very communities these patients hate," Ashley said and began giving Gerald the catalogue of evidence she had gathered all week.

She told him about the sick pigs, the blood rituals, and the probable sexual relationships revealed.

"It sounds like Burt Williams does more than the charity work he claims to do in Atlanta," Gerald said. "I have not gotten to know Betty Ann Williams well enough to find out any more than that her husband traveled there recently."

"At least you got that," Ashley said. "Oh, and then Sophia saw the exchange in the hallway between Burt Williams and Ronnie Lynch. And Ronnie talked to Thomas about how upset he was that Burt Williams, alias R. E. Lee, would not talk with him when he called him later that day."

"It would be helpful to know what goes on in that Atlanta bar," Gerald said.

"Well, Brugge, Fred and Thomas took a field trip down there today. They're off the weekend."

"Really?" Gerald asked.

"Yup. They thought it would be a good idea to check it out, especially since Mr. Wilson mentioned to Fred that he goes to JD's in Atlanta every time he's there for charity work, and Ronnie dropped that napkin from that bar with R. E. Lee's name and number on it. Of course, we had that clue from Ronnie's secret service man originally, didn't we?"

"Sure did. Ashley, we are covering Fred and Thomas' expenses, correct?"

"Of course. I offered them hourly wages because they are working, after all, and car rental, hotel, food, and drinks."

"Good, good," Gerald said.

Then Ashley told Gerald about how Sam Smith's pig in Alabama and George Johnson's in Georgia came from the same farm in North Carolina.

"How on earth did they find out that?" Gerald asked.

"Well, Jack said Reba Smith's daughter told her mother last evening to tell us the name of the farm in case the pig got her parents sick and anyone else." Ashley continued, "And then today Dan found out from Mrs. Johnson that her nine-year old grandson saw Mr. Johnson and some other men place the pig's blood on each other's foreheads after killing it before Christmas, just like Mrs. Smith's daughter saw her father do."

"It's amazing, the details the nurses got from them. What on earth made Mrs. Johnson tell Dan about what her grandson saw?"

Ashley explained how close Dan had become with Mrs. Johnson throughout the week, especially before her husband was ventilated. Dan had told Ashley that Mrs. Johnson was starting to get scared as her husband's pneumonia got worse throughout the week, and she thought she should tell the nurse everything she knew.

Ashley added," Oh, and a friend of Mrs. Johnson's back in Darien called her yesterday and said her own husband got real sick too with a strange pneumonia and diarrhea but wasn't in the hospital like her husband was. Turns out, George Johnson gave that man one of those pigs.

"Dan told us during report about an hour ago how he asked Mrs. Johnson if she remembered the name of the farm where Georgie got the pig because it might be helpful if any other people got sick."

"Well, well, Ashley. It's starting to sound like a zoonotic transmission of some virus. And if it is indeed a virus that jumped from pig to human, it looks like it is sexually trans-mitted between humans. Maybe that's why Reba Smith and Betty Ann Williams and even Ronnie Lynch are sick. What a wealth of information, Ashley! So, what's the name of the farm?"

"Porky's in Clinton, North Carolina. I thought poor Sophia, though, was going to faint. She's on duty tonight."

"Why's that?"

"She turned pale as a ghost after Dan told us the name. Then, she asked him, 'Did you say Porky's?' "Dan said, 'That's what Mrs. J told me. Yup. Are you OK, Sophia?'"

"Sophia said, 'That's my father-in-law's farm.' I got chills up my spine, Gerald."

"Wow, Ashley. All this is starting to feel like an episode of *House*."

"I agree, Brugge! And I actually can because that was one of my faves when I was a teenager."

"I'm just pleased we both know the same cultural reference."

Ashley laughed.

PART 3

NOT AGAIN

Fred and Thomas were ready to go. When Fred told Linda about Atlanta, she suggested an early breakfast to send them off.

Linda and Thomas had just ordered some coffee. Thomas was asking her as much as he could about San Francisco, how she got there and why she stayed. And Linda was intrigued by Thomas' choice to leave behind his medical school training.

"I understand why you wanted to be a nurse back then, Thomas. The doctors were mainly worried about finding the cause, thankfully, and then the cure while we were worried about them dying with dignity and feeling some tenderness, any crumb of compassion, before they left their misery behind."

"Hey, everyone," Fred said and sat down. "I should warn you, Thomas, Linda Washington doesn't open up to just anyone, and from what I can see she may be on her way with you. It'll take some time, though, the layers are deep."

"Indeed, they are, Frederick. It's something really. I did not realize until I started caring for these patients now, working with fellow nurses who served back then, how much cashmere, so to speak, I've wrapped myself in all these years just to keep my memories comfortably tucked away, well suppressed really. But it's starting to feel now like I need a different material, like silk perhaps, to give them a little air."

"I like that, Thomas," Linda said.

"I do, too," Fred said. "However you want to describe what we AIDS nurses have done, had to do, still do, in order to keep our experiences hidden away enough, just enough, to keep functioning in the world."

"So boys, how long will you be in Atlanta?" Linda asked.

"I'm hoping we find out what we need tonight. I want to stop in Clayton also where that one guy I've been taking care of lives," Fred said.

"Where's that?" Linda asked.

Fred said it looked about one and a half to two hours north of Atlanta on the map. They could reach Alvin in Wonderland around 5:00 P.M., just in time for dinner, in the South anyway.

"Isn't that one of Rumpel's places?" Linda asked.

"Sure is. Not that my patient knew that. He just kept going on and on about the Mexicans and Salvadorans leaking out of the place. We thought we should check it out."

"If you can stomach giving your money to one of his businesses," Linda added.

"Well, it's not our money is it? The trip's on the NHC, really the VP. Anyway, Thomas and I thought it might be worth it to see how many immigrants are working there and how they are treated. It might give us some idea about how much worse this country is going to treat non-whites in the future.

"I mean hell, Linda, as you know, my husband, who is no

longer recognized as my husband, is Chinese-American and I'm starting to really worry about the Chinese part."

"I would love to marry my current partner, Linda. I've discussed that with Frederick. I finally found the person I just cannot do without and gay marriage is illegal once again. And my partner is Black and Vietnamese. I share Frederick's concerns."

"He must be beautiful," Linda said.

"He is," Thomas said and pulled up his picture on his phone. "This is An Tyrone, a fellow NP," Thomas said.

"Fred, wasn't that our patient's name, from the early years? The one who drank ...."

"Yeah, Linda. An Trán, from the Tenderloin," Fred said and began the story as they ordered breakfast.

An Trán came to the AIDS Ward at Bay City General in early 1985. His stage name was Chau.

"An was his male name," Fred said.

"I know, Frederick. Chau is a female Vietnamese name that means 'pearl'," Thomas said.

"Yes, but as you must know then, An means 'peace,' something that poor boy never got any of as An or Chau," Fred said.

The Trán family made it to San Francisco in 1976 after the war in Vietnam officially ended. An was ten and remembered all of the details. The escape boat was nowhere big or sturdy enough to sustain the three families who jumped on board, ready to leave behind their now communist country.

An used to tell the nurses how grateful his family was to the U.S. Navy for transporting hundreds upon hundreds of them to California on a "big sea spaceship," as he called it.

San Francisco was the natural choice for An's parents because his mother's sister had fled there from American military infected Vietnam years before. An's auntie always wrote letters inviting them to settle in San Francisco where they could eat delicious food from their homeland, plus American burgers and pizza, while enjoying the cooler climate and looking out at the rust-beamed bridge that "just floated in the air," she always told them.

And settle they did in Auntie Chau's one bedroom apartment in the Tenderloin district on Larkin Street. There were nine of them in that little box: Auntie Chau and her three boys. Her husband died from tuberculosis during their boat trip to the USA. And there was An, his two sisters, and his parents. All of them worked in Auntie Chau's restaurant.

"An told me," Fred said, "he chose his aunt's name for the stage and for the woman he really wanted to be."

Linda added, "An would tell us his Auntie Chau was a caring, beautiful woman outside and in."

"She was the only one who visited him in the end," Fred said.

"Until she could not," Linda said.

"What happened?" Thomas was engaged in a way he normally was not.

The waitress placed the tray of pastry assortments on the table next to the French pressed coffee and asked if she could top off anyone's cup.

"Thank you, yes," Fred said and chose one. "Is this a wife cake?"

"It is. Our pastry chef loves to make them and we love to eat them. He's Chinese," the waitress said.

"I do, too. Always have them back home," Fred said.

The waitress smiled after pouring Fred's coffee.

"Hey, Linda. An always ordered wife cakes from that one shop on Stockton Street, remember?"

"I do, but he never ate them," Linda said.

"An had more of a mental appetite for them, I assume," Thomas said.

"Yes, as you know, so many of our patients experienced that, the memory of the taste of their favorite foods. An could hardly eat anything. His stomach was blocked by that awful cancer," Linda said.

Fred admitted An Trán on a stormy night in January 1985. Fred remembered it was January because the thunder and lightning were so unusual for that time of year, and he had been struggling as a first year RN to maintain healthy boundaries with patients, like An.

One of the night shift nurses had called out sick and the supervisor could not, would not really, transfer another nurse to the AIDS Ward. Fred, who was supposed to be off duty at 7:30 P.M., volunteered to work until 11:00 P.M. when the patients supposedly were more settled for the night and the empty beds would be filled.

An had been sick for a while but Chau still attracted late night crowds at La Cage until the projectile vomiting started to interfere with her sets.

Auntie Chau made it to most of her nephew's shows, especially after the rest of the family had stopped welcoming An into her home. An's auntie also made big pots of noodles and veggies she left backstage for her nephew to share with Golden Kate Bridge, An's fellow performer and partner with whom he shared a one bedroom room in the hotel for entertainers on Eddy Street, not far from the Trán family in the Tenderloin.

An had a feeling the vomiting might be a sign of the "San Francisco flu," as he and his friends referred to the new illness. He often thought about those nights when he had to do whatever he could to survive before landing the steady stream of shows at La Cage in the Tenderloin.

The endoscopy performed shortly after An's admission to Bay City General revealed Burkitt's lymphoma. Linda said to

Fred now, "I was on the day An came back to the floor from the procedure.

"The doctor who did it said to me, 'I've never seen anything like it. This guy is barely twenty and has a tumor the size of a softball blocking his duodenum. I couldn't even pass the damn scope through his pyloric sphincter. But I got a biopsy of the edge of the thing. What the hell's happening to these freaks?'"

"They always had the most charming names for our patients, didn't they," Thomas said.

Fred then talked about the surgeon who was consulted and how he would not even consider removing An's tumor because of the AIDS, even though that could not be confirmed until the HIV antibody test became available a few months later.

"They ordered chemotherapy, really toxic shit. An got even sicker, and it sure as hell did not work," Fred said.

"I don't remember the chemo, Fred. But what I do remember is An lost someone he loved just about every week," Linda said.

An's partner, Kate, was admitted to the ICU at Bay City General after one week of singing and dancing with temps above 102 degrees and shortness of breath that set in after only one chorus of "I Will Survive."

La Cage's manager called An to tell him Kate also left him "high and dry," he said. "It's just one of you after another these days." The nurses wheeled An down to the ICU for one last visit.

Then An's parents visited him, but only once. They thought their son really might be dying just from cancer. But about an hour into their visit they started to suspect AIDS after seeing the other young patients and their visitors.

Hanh, An's older sister, visited the following week, but just scolded him the whole time for bringing disgrace to the family.

"You could've just hidden your feelings about men, about wanting to be a woman," she told him crying.

An's younger sister, Binh, visited him every couple of nights. She never cared about who An loved or who he wanted to be. But when Binh could see An's bones stretching the surface of his skin like the stuffing in a thin-walled wonton wrap, thanks to the HIV and the lymphoma stealing all of his body's energy and steering him onto the straight path to death, she could not bring herself to return.

"My An, my Chau, I say my goodbyes. I cannot see you no more. I love you," Binh said. That was early April 1985.

Then Fred talked about An's own Auntie Chau being the only one left who came to visit him. One night she brought him a wife cake she made, even though the nurses told her he never ate them.

"That wife cake was the last night she came in," Fred said. "I remember his auntie sitting next to him in his bed encouraging him to take just one bite. And he did. And then another. Then he ate the whole thing. She kissed him goodbye and said she would see him the following night. I think that was in May,"

"It was, Fred," Linda said. "I remember because my Anthony, my son, was still alive and well in Dallas then."

Fred said he was on duty the next day when An's younger sister called to tell him Auntie Chau was run over by the F line on her way back home to the Tenderloin after visiting An. An's sister said the conductor told her that her auntie just walked in front of the streetcar without even looking.

"She must have been so distraught, Fred. He was so sick. He barely weighed 60 pounds," Linda said.

Fred shook his head and continued on to the end. When Auntie Chau did not come in at 6:00 P.M., her regular time, An got out of bed for the first time in a week and sat in the chair by the window. He sat there staring down at Folsom Street, waiting to see her until the sky turned black.

"We were so damn busy that night. I should've been home hours ago but I wanted to check in on An one more time."

"I couldn't believe it. He was in bed sitting up but his head was bent over his chest. There was blood everywhere. It took me a minute to figure out where it was coming from. Then I saw it was still dripping from his mouth.

"I kicked the bottle of empty beach on the floor as I approached the head of his bed, realizing then what he had done. 'An, An, Chau,' I yelled as I shook his shoulders and placed a cloth beneath his chin. 'Why did you?'

"He could barely get the words out. 'I am clean now,' he said. 'No more AIDS. Auntie might forgive me.'

"Then he was gone."

"What a dreadful experience, Frederick, for that young boy and for you," Thomas said.

"Indeed, it was, Thomas," Linda said.

Fred just sat there, staring at the untouched wife cake on his plate.

JUNE 11, 2021, 1:00 P.M.
National Health Center, Respiratory Unit, Staff Lounge

Margarita was thanking Cal, again, for switching assignments with her so she could take care of Betty Ann Williams, even though she knew it would be a hard shift because the patient still required frequent and intense monitoring for the Dopamine drip keeping her kidneys going.

But at least Margarita felt safe with her. The patient would comment on how sweet Margarita was and what a good nurse she was, and then always manage to slip in that she could not believe she was American with her "dark roasted coffee skin."

Margarita was able to place those remarks in her box for the shift, though.

"No problem girl," Cal said. "Ms. Reba is easy breezy and ready for discharge tomorrow. That Wilson is God awful, though, with his constant nastiness talking about Mexicans all the time. Of course, he's not too thrilled with the likes of me either, but I can handle him."

"Yeah, Cal, that's what I've heard all the other nurses say too. And in report this morning, I heard Mr. Wilson had mentioned to Fred that an Alvin in Wonderland had hurt his business down in Georgia.

"The mention of that place turns my blood mucho frío. I can't place those feelings away for a minute, let alone the whole shift."

"Hey, why's that, Margarita?" Dan who just came in asked.

Margarita Ramirez told Dan and Cal all about her family so they would understand. Her parents came to the United States from Tijuana, Mexico, in 1996. Her father was a professional chef and her mother ran a successful B&B serving her husband's fusion Mexican Baja cuisine to a primarily international clientele.

Her parents wanted to experience the U.S.A, though, after hearing friends and relatives talk about even more opportunities there, especially in the eastern states, like Delaware, where casinos started popping up in 1995.

They got work permits. Margarita's mother took a job running a coffee shop in a Dover casino and her father was offered the sous chef position in a Michelin star restaurant there that the owner wanted to turn into two stars with her father's talents.

Margarita was born not long after they arrived. By the time she reached high school, her parents opened their own restaurant in the casino, Ramirez Bistro, where she worked as a teenager, but her heart yearned for a career in nursing.

It was hard for Margarita's parents when she moved to the D.C. area to take her first nursing job at the NHC, but she spoke to them often and went home every month or two. That's why she knew what she did about Alvin in Wonderland.

One of these places had opened last year in the Dover casino. All of the Alvin in Wonderlands adopted the cuisine of the most popular restaurants in their vicinity, and Ramirez Bistro was one of them, offering cheaper versions of it, in every way, and entertainment.

"It's what the entertainment is that I can't ignore, guys. I have cousins who work in the one back home. They make minimum wage without any benefits. But the worst part is my people are made to be the entertainment."

"You mean this dinner theatre like forces Mexicans to dance and sing?" Dan asked.

"I wish that was it. We wish. No, people from the crowd at each show take shots at them," Margarita said.

"You mean they like make them the object of jokes?" Dan said.

"No, Dan, I mean Mexicans who have been caught at the borders are literally shot."

"Lordy be. Just when you think that president couldn't possibly do anything worse," Cal said.

JUNE 11, 2021, 6:00 P.M.
Alvin in Wonderland, Clayton, Georgia

Fred and Thomas had arrived less than an hour ago. They could not believe the lines. The doors closed at 5:30 P.M. and would not open again until 7:00 P.M. for the last show of the night.

The man selling tickets asked them when they reached the window, "Spectator or actor?"

"Well, let's see. Spectator, of course," Thomas said.

"That'll be $50 a piece."

"How much to be an actor?" Fred asked.

"Regular $100. Supreme $200."

"We'll take two spectators. Thank you," Thomas said and paid.

Both of them could not wait to find out what a regular actor was, let alone a supreme one, and why anyone would pay so much to be one.

The dinner was bad. Fred had always wanted to see and taste the South. Thomas liked Savannah, Georgia, and spent time there with An so he assured Fred good fried chicken was crispy not rubbery, and good collards coated your tongue with pork soaked goodness and not the sugar substitute taste lingering in these greens.

"You would think the bourbon, at least, would be top shelf," Fred said.

"This tastes dreadful, indeed. Just as well, Frederick, it looks like our show is about to begin," Thomas said.

The host asked the regular actors to join him on stage. There were three of them.

"Those guys don't look like actors, Thomas. They look like beer guzzling rednecks," Fred said.

"Indeed," Thomas said.

The host began to call out names of Mexicans who joined the stage one by one:

"Juan Gonzales, San Diego, California border.

"Tito Velazquez, El Paso, Texas border.

"Veronica Menendez, Sonora, Arizona border.

The host then handed a bow and arrow to "regular actor #1" and instructed Juan Gonzales to stand in a circle painted on the floor about twenty-four feet away.

The host spoke through the microphone, "You should have stayed home. America's arms have been open for too long to the tired and poor of Mexico.

"Take aim," the host instructed the actor. "Shoot."

Juan Gonzales fell to the stage floor after the arrow penetrated his chest. The same fate awaited the other two contestants, as the host called the victims.

Fred's phone was vibrating in his pocket. He took it out and read the text from Cal, "Are you and Thomas making it to that dinner theatre? Margarita filled us in on the entertainment. Not good, honey."

Moments later, the host called supreme actors #1 and #2 to the stage after the three bodies were dragged away. A small guillotine had been rolled onto the stage before the curtain parted for the audience.

"Can you believe this, Thomas?" Fred whispered.

"I am absolutely speechless," Thomas replied.

Two more Mexican names were called out. They were escorted to the stage this time by a big bouncer-looking white man with a swastika tattooed on his neck.

As the blade swooshed down to meet Chico Rivera's neck, Fred texted back Cal," It's awful here, Cali girl. We made it for the Wild Wild West dinner show and now the Reign of Terror dessert. I'll call you soon. Can't wait to leave."

June 11, 2021, 8:30 P.M.
JD's, Atlanta, Georgia

Both of them were looking forward to at least one good drink, hoping Mr. Wilson was right about the alcohol in this place. Fred and Thomas ordered two bourbons on the rocks.

"Keep your hoods lowered," Fred repeated the sign at the entrance. "What the hell does that mean? Is this really a Klan hangout?"

"I don't know, Frederick. I can't say I've ever been in one before, but that over there doesn't make me doubt that it is," Thomas said pointing to a huge cloth Confederate flag covering most of the wall.

"Well, you certainly would not see the crowd in here at a Pride parade," Fred said.

"Certainly not," Thomas said with a little smile.

The bourbon was good. Fred had to admit it was the best he ever had. They ordered one more round to help dull the memory of the lynching performance they witnessed just a few hours ago.

Country music was playing with some old Rock n' Roll every few songs. The flat screen TV near the front of the bar had on the news station that only covered Rumpel's activities, businesses, family, and daily speeches delivered in front of the Lincoln Memorial where the camera made Rumpel look bigger than the sitting, dignified President of the United States whose stature reflected his role in navigating this nation through the murky waters of institutionalized racism and the Civil War.

The TV screen in the back of the bar showed hooded and unhooded KKK members hanging Blacks, Latinos, and white people from trees with the caption every time a white man was on the rope: "This faggot's skin color did not save him."

Halfway through their second drinks, a handsome middle-aged man approached the young guy sitting a few seats away from Fred at the bar.

"Hi there, fella. You must be Carpetbagger Carl," the man said.

"How'd you guess?" the young man said.

"You're not a regular in here, so I just figured. I'm R.E. Lee. How's about a drink?"

"Sure thing."

"Hey, Jimmy," Burt Williams said to the bartender. "Two regulars would fix us right quick."

Burt led the boy to a booth in the back of the bar.

"Did you hear that, Frederick? That's R.E. Lee. I never imagined we would actually see him here," Thomas said. "That guy gets around."

"Did he see you? You took care of his wife didn't you, the other day when he visited?" Fred asked.

"I don't think he saw me then. He only stayed a few hours at the hospital and spent most of his time off the floor. I only got a glimpse of him leaving that day, Frederick."

"This is unreal," Fred said.

"Frederick, can you stay on the lookout? I will keep my back to him just in case. Tell me what you see."

Burt Williams had a lot in common with this young man, Bobby Taylor, a 23-year-old Business degree graduate from Baltimore who could not find a job. He told Burt now, "That city just wants those people to fill up any open position."

Bobby, alias Carpetbagger Carl, had always thought of Maryland as the North and felt like he had much more in common with good old Southern boys. He found Burt Williams in the chat room of "Blinded by the White" in search of some conversations with white supremacists.

"Thomas," Fred said. "They left."

"I didn't see them go through the front door."

"They did not. They walked hand in hand behind that curtain back there," Fred said.

Thomas turned around to look and said, "Unreal."

JUNE 11, 202, 11:00 P.M.
Here to Stay Bar, Atlanta, Georgia

"Cali girl was right about this place, Thomas. Upbeat, good menu and music, and nice eye candy," Fred said.

"I needed a good gay bar after that place, Frederick. Or shall I say a good 'openly' gay bar with all types."

"Yeah, All white can be so boring," Fred said.

"And dangerous in a place like that. Sooo, Frederick. Tell me about the first man of your dreams, the one who called you by your proper name."

"How do you know he was my first, Thomas?"

"You mentioned, during the first shift we worked together, that you had not been called Frederick in a long time. I figured it must have been someone really special in your life."

"Yes. Winston."

"Where is he now?"

"In Chicago. *The Bohemian Cemetery.*

Fred told Thomas about when he first met Winston in the summer of 1979. Fred was 16 years old when he discovered Boystown, the first official gay neighborhood in Chicago, and his refuge from his awful teen years in Montgomery, Illinois, a small town less than one hour away from the big city.

Fred's father had worked his whole life in Montgomery's main industry, a tractor plant. At least he did until the massive heart attack he had at 38 years old.

Fred was only ten when his father died. Then his mother got really religious. The preacher at the Pentecostal church she started to attend started preying on her vulnerability and the handsome pension transferred to her from the plant after her husband's death.

Preacher Travis also preyed on young Fred. Fred had a feeling he liked boys when his school friends started talking about all of the cute girls on the playground and Fred did not share in their interest.

But Fred sure was not interested in the inappropriate advances made by Preacher Travis after his mother married him. Travis demanded Fred call him "Dad," but Fred never called him anything but "Preacher" followed by a strong "Ha." He fought off Travis anytime he came into his room, thanks to the tall muscular frame he inherited from his father.

At fifteen, Fred got a job as a busboy in a nice Chicago steakhouse. Fred now told Thomas that his mother was not happy about him working in Chicago but Fred convinced her it was just fine because the bus took him there in an hour and the money was good.

The waiters started taking him along to Jim's in Boystown the following year. It was the best bar for good music, only if you were sixteen, and drinks, only if you were eighteen. And Jim's owner enforced these rules for the patrons inside while trying to keep the police out by padding the walls and windows to prevent any neighborhood complaints about noise or light, which always invited a raid.

Winston Church was one of the regulars at Jim's and knew Fred ever since he started coming in with the other wait staff. Fred knew Winston was eight years older than him but Fred liked Winston's youthful approach to life, especially captured in his fashion designs.

Shortly after they met, Winston told Fred his last name was short for the "best damn prime minister England ever had" and had nothing to do with any house of worship that "turned me away long ago just for being me."

Winston was the first at Jim's to buy Fred a beer when he turned eighteen and the first to ask him out. They fell in love not long after that and Fred moved in with him.

But after two years Fred could not take sharing Winston any longer with other men they "picked up together," as Winston saw it. That's when Fred told him about the nursing school in San Francisco that accepted him and offered to cover his three-year tuition in February 1981.

"Why nursing, Frederick?" Winston asked him. "You have a great job at the steakhouse. You have moved yourself up to head waiter after only two years."

"Well, I can't imagine being one in ten years, or twenty, for sure. I need something more stimulating, Winston. Nursing is trying to take in more men, and quite frankly I find I want to talk to my customers more and more about their lives, their problems, and not just if they want their steaks medium rare, or well done, which no one should ever ask for anyway." They both laughed.

They made love for the last time, just the two of them, the night before Fred moved to San Francisco at the end of May. He thought he could enjoy the summer there, waiting tables to make some money, until the hospital diploma program at Bay City General Hospital began its classes in early August.

About a week after Fred found a room to rent in the Castro, he walked by a newsstand and could not help buying *The Chronicle* that June 5, 1981. The front-page story announced five men in L.A. who had a rare type of pneumonia and all of them were homosexuals. A chill ran up Fred's spine. Winston, he thought.

"So, Frederick, I assume Winston died of AIDS back

then?" Thomas asked as the theme night disco music pumped in the background of the bar.

"You would think. I sure did. I still saw him when I went home to Chicago but over the years that was less and less. I always asked him if he got tested and he would say, 'Now Frederick, you know me. There's no need for that. When my time's up, it's up.'"

Fred fast forwarded to 1993. He had been working on the AIDS Ward at Bay City General for almost nine years when Winston called him on Valentine's day. He did not sound well at all.

Fred told Li Yong, his new boyfriend, that he needed to go to Chicago. By the time Fred landed on a delayed flight at the blizzard-enveloped airport, the nurse from Ward 222, the AIDS Unit at County Hospital, had called to tell Fred to hurry.

Winston was in a semi-private room. "Thank goodness," Fred had said out loud walking down the hallway past several four-bedded ones. Then he thought about how fortunate they were in San Francisco to have private rooms for all of their patients.

"He looked so awful, Thomas," Fred said, sipping some wine while trying to not let any tears fill up in his eyes.

When Fred found Winston's room, he walked over to the bed near the window. "That can't be right." He went back out to look at the door sign to make sure the window bed was 4B and not 4A.

Fred then lifted up the sleeping man's brown stick of an arm that had replaced the developed musculature from all the cloth Winston had cut and the feeding of it with such ease into the sewing machine time after time, and the dance of his own single magic needle topping off every one of his sartorial masterpieces with his threaded signature.

The name bracelet slipped off of Winston's wrist when Fred rested his arm back on the bed. This wraith, this collection of bones clutching onto the remaining cobwebbed skin, was indeed Fred's first love, the vibrant creator of Churchwear.

"Frederick," Winston opened his eyes. "I am so glad you are here. Thank you."

Fred could not leave him. He was not in love with him any longer but he loved him. "No one had been around to see him," the nurse had told Fred. No one at all visited Winston Church. All the lovers, the department store buyers, the fans, everyone who would have given almost anything for a Churchwear original, were absent.

Fred knew it would be anywhere from a few days to a few weeks. He called Linda Washington, now his immediate supervisor and said he had to stay. "Of course," she said. She knew. There was no one else to walk the last mile with them, and then carry them until they were forced to leave much sooner than they ever could have imagined.

The virus probably crossed into Winston's brain. It was hard to tell because he laughed most of the time instead of screaming or crying like other patients had done.

He laughed, even when a few nights later, Fred was cleaning up what he thought was a large, bloody bowel movement caused by the Burkitt's lymphoma strangling his large intestine, but turned out to be Winston's spleen, pancreas, and gall bladder coming out one by one.

Fred asked the nurse to give Winston some morphine. He could not imagine Winston did not feel pain somewhere deep in his gut from the tissue and blood he just lost, and maybe in his head where the feeling had just not registered as pain.

And the laughing never stopped, making it so hard for Fred to comfort Winston with soft words and touches. Kathy, Winston's night nurse that night, made sure he had morphine every hour and Haldol every three to at least dull the maniacal sound bordering on heckling.

When the laughing stopped the next day, the breathing was not far behind. Winston was only 38 years old, just like Fred's own father, and no one in this world cared about him except Fred.

Fred wrote an elegy for him and paid a hefty sum to print it as his obituary in Chicago's big newspaper. He had a memorial service for Winston back home in San Francisco. Li Yong helped Fred with every detail and told his future husband, "If you loved him, Fred, he must have been a good one."

JUNE 12, 2021, 8:00 P.M.
Giovanni's, Crystal City, Va.

Sophia said to Dan, Sura, and Linda, really only Dan, "It seems so weird, all of this coming from my own family."

"How long has your father-in-law had his farm?" Dan asked sipping the one glass of chianti he allowed himself with dinner every evening.

Dan found this restaurant during a long walk, he told the ladies when they arrived, and thought it would be a step or two above the pizzeria he spent a lot of his time in.

"A long time. It's been in the Abbott family since my husband's grandfather bought it in the 1940s," Sophia said.

"He named it after Porky Pig, right Sophia?" Dan asked.

"Sure did. His favorite Looney Tunes character, who he imitated any chance he could get, I've been told by the Abbott men."

"That's cute. I ask because when Jack was telling us about Mrs. S. not remembering the name of the farm where her husband got the pig, she said it was named after an old Looney

Tunes character, and Ashley and Margarita didn't know what that was," Dan said.

"I'm not surprised at all. My niece and nephew, Maria and Mario, are in their early twenties and they do not get any references we make about anything earlier than 1980. Even that year is too early for them sometimes. They did not know who Rock Hudson was or that he was one of the first famous people to die from AIDS."

"Yeah, I got 'em that age in my family too. They don't know him either. I sat them down once and showed them a movie or two, though."

"No children of your own, Dan?" Sophia asked as Sura and Linda talked to each other only, like matchmakers chaperoning a first date.

"Nah, I like 'em alright but never wanted my own."

"Me, neither," Sophia said.

"Did your husband want children, Sophia?"

"Never did. He had his own causes to nurture, too. He represented people who no one else did. Worked a lot with the CLO."

"He's a lawyer then. Nice," Dan said.

"Was," Sophia said.

Dan knew from Linda that Sophia was a widow when he had asked about her, but he did not want to be too forward now.

"He's dead, Dan. Since 2008. Ricky had a sharp mind and a good heart."

"Sounds like it, Sophia. It's nice you've kept up your relationship with his father."

"I don't see him as much as I'd like, especially since I moved to Italy a few years ago. I encourage him to visit since he's alone. My mother-in-law, Emma, died a few years after Ricky did. Ovarian cancer."

"I hate that one but I'm not an oncology nurse, only treated the cancers our AIDS patients got. But I sure wish I didn't know anything about that one."

"I agree completely. My grandmother and mother-in-law were enough for me," Sophia said. She knew from Sura that Dan was widowed, and she was thinking now that this cancer might have been the culprit.

Then Dan said, "For me, it was my wife. Naomi. She died in 2010. Her family didn't want to keep me around after that, though."

"Why not?" Sophia asked.

"They were pretty Jewish. Never accepted me because I would not convert. That was back in L.A. I used to tell 'em before Naomi and I got married in like 2000, 'No offense, Mr. and Mrs. Levy, but my Italian Catholic family would disown me. They practically have anyway, ever since I told 'em I wasn't so sure about God.'

"Boy, they looked at me then, like I was from outer space. I said, 'It's hard to believe when you've watched one young person after another leave this world in a state of complete misery, and for like years'."

"So true, Dan. Well, my family tolerated Ricky being a Methodist but he was not religious at all. Now my in-laws at first thought I was a little 'too ethnic,' as they liked to put it. But they actually grew to really like the Italian and Puerto Rican dishes I made during the holidays.

"Catholicism was acceptable to them, at least it was Christian, but that never stopped my father-in-law from commenting about the saints, all the statutes, and of course, the priests.

"'If they allowed them to fool around a little, maybe they wouldn't be picking on those boys all the time,' Tucker would say on more than one occasion."

Dan laughed.

Sophia continued. "I've never really discussed my atheism with my father-in-law and I sure never did with my father when he was alive. My mother understands why it happened but she does not approve."

"Ditto for mine," Dan said. "So, Sophia, have you called your father-in-law to give him a heads up? It sounds like the NHC or the CDB or both are going to contact him soon."

"I'm working up to it, Dan. Tucker knows I've been back in the States. I talked to him before I left Florence and told him I was coming to see the Quilt. As you know, everything has happened so fast since then so I never updated him on being here and working and all that."

"How old is he now, Sophia?"

"Mid-80s."

"I know you know but it might be easier for him to hear it from you rather than getting some kind of official call scaring the hell out of him."

"It would take a lot to do that to Tucker Abbott, old farmer that he is now. But you're so right. I just hate to always be the bearer of bad news."

"You mean like when your husband got sick, Sophia?"

"Yeah. But I guess I haven't given Tucker any news like that in a long time."

"This might not be such bad news, Sophia. I mean we found what looks like the source of this new illness after only one week. And your father-in-law isn't sick, right?"

"He wasn't at the end of May."

Sophia sipped her cappuccino and took a bite of cannoli. "That's good. Not Arthur Avenue good. But good."

"Nothing like cannoli from up there. Inside the States, anyway, as you know," Dan said.

"I do need to call him. I'm remembering something he told me last Christmas," Sophia said and stood to leave.

"Thank you so much, Dan, for the nice dinner and conversation."

Dan took her hand and kissed it. Sophia smiled.

"Danny, she is a sweet girl," Linda told him after she watched Sophia walk out the front door.

"She is, Dan, always has been," Sura said.

"You two have a lot in common," Linda said.

"A whole lot of death, for sure, both professional and personal."

"There's a lot of life there too," Sura said.

June 13, 2021, 6:00 P.M.
Crystal Nightingale Hotel, Crystal City, Va.

Sophia waited all day to call Tucker Abbott. She did not want to disturb his farming duties, she kept telling herself that anyway. Earlier in the day she enjoyed a Botticelli exhibit at the *National Museum of Art* and a superb lunch at a French restaurant.

But now, at this time, she knew Tucker would be done with his dinner, chicken and noodles like he usually made because he never could bring himself to eat any of the pigs he raised.

"Good evening," Tucker said when he picked up the phone and walked across the kitchen stretching the long cord so he could wash the dishes.

"Tuck, it's me, Sophia."

"How are you darl'n? How'd you do with that Quilt? Must've teared you right up. Can't understand why it has to be the last time to see it."

"No one with any sense understands that one, Tucker."

"That's one for the history books to answer, for sure."

"The Quilt was hard, Tucker. But I still had my sister Terri with me then."

"Terri. That's right. Hope she's well."

"She is. Thank you. I also was with some of the nurses I worked with back then."

"Like that Serena. The Holocaust survivor. The one I met at Ricky's funeral."

"Yes. It's Sura, though, and her family got out of Germany before they were sent to the death camps."

"Well, she sure did survive then, didn't she? She's very nice. Proper."

"Tucker, we old AIDS nurses were asked to work temporarily at the National Health Center."

"Why's that, Sophia?"

"There's been a new sickness in a population no one wants to care for. And we needed to get some answers in order to find the source quickly."

"Well look at that, you're right on the front lines once again. What's this illness, Sophia?"

"Some people get really bad diarrhea. Some develop purple lesions and kidney failure. Others get pneumonia or some combination of all that."

"That doesn't sound so good. So, what's the cause, Sophia, that all of you helped to find?"

"This is where it gets really interesting, Tucker. It appears to come from pigs."

"Not too unusual. Swine flu is, too, but you know better than I do about all that."

"Well, this isn't flu or any other virus we know about yet. All the patients we've been taking care of, though, bought, or were affiliated with someone, it turns out, who bought some pigs from your farm."

Tucker was matter of fact in his response. "When did they buy 'em, Sophia?"

"We've traced them all back to the end of last October."

"Well, I'll be. I believe I had a litter then a little less robust than normal. Told the guys I sold 'em to they weren't acting right on account of the heat. That's what I thought then anyway."

"What could have been wrong with them, Tucker? And forgive me, how many are in a litter again? I know I should remember."

"Ten, if it's a good one. You know I vaccinate all my pigs, never miss one, especially for that porcine virus. It'll make pigs real sick if they get it."

"Do you remember who bought that litter, Tucker?"

"Sure do. Couldn't forget them if I tried. They all wore hoods."

"You mean white ones?"

"Yup. Klan hoods, to be sure. And they all had the same letters on their license plates."

"What was that?" Sophia asked him, but had a feeling she knew the answer.

"JD."

"Tucker, do you remember last Christmas when we talked you told me you had been having loose bowels?"

"Come to think of it, I do now, Sophia."

"Did you ever get any sicker?"

"Nope. On and off for about a month or two. Then it was gone."

"Interesting," Sophia said. "You fed that litter you sold to those men or did your farm hand?"

"You know me, Sophia. I can't help but tend to a new litter myself. I love to watch 'em grow. Can't do that so much anymore since I have to sell 'em so young on account of the soy bean expense.

"Are you thinking I might've had a mild case of what my pigs had from handling them, Sophia?"

"Yes, not that I know that much about how viruses jump to us from animals."

"How did it jump to the people you've been caring for?"

"I'm not so sure I want to say too much about all that yet, Tucker."

"Do the doctors need to test me and my farm?"

"I believe so. Dr. Brugge, who I have been working with, indicated that much yesterday morning before I got off duty. He needs to talk to the CDB, you know the Central Disease Bureau in Atlanta, tomorrow."

"Well, hell, Sophia. I'm right here. So are my pigs until they're sold. Just don't ask me to come all the way up there into that craziness, or even to Atlanta. Terrible driving there."

"We would never ask you to do that. Thank you so much. Love you. See you soon, Tucker."

"Love you right back, darl'n. I hope so."

June 14, 2021, 7:30 A.M.
National Health Center, Respiratory Unit, Staff Lounge

The nurses going off and coming on duty, and especially Gerald Brugge and Ashley Smith, could not wait to hear about Fred and Thomas' trip to Georgia.

Cal could not help herself after Thomas shared the Burt Williams part of the story. "Whooeee! Ms. Betty's boo sure does get around!"

All of them were shocked when Fred described the "entertainment" at Alvin in Wonderland's, except for Cal. "I told you all about what Margarita said. That shit is bad, bad, bad."

Then Ashley told them about Sophia calling her early this morning to let her know she spoke with her father-in-law last night.

"Mr. Tucker Abbott, Sophia told me, confirmed that he sold a litter of pigs to five men last October. He remembers them because they wore hoods during their purchase."

"Holy shit," Bridgette, who did not want to end her shift quite yet, said.

"How many comprises a litter?" Thomas asked.

"Ten, sweetie, ten," Cal chimed in.

"Plus, Sophia told me her father-in-law remembered all of their license plates having the same letters," Ashley continued.

"Let me guess," Fred said. "JD."

"Yup, that's what Mr. Abbott told her. But she said her father-in-law thought it was a reference to the type of liquor they liked to drink," Ashley said.

Gerald laughed a little and then said," Do we really know the meaning? It could be Jack Daniels."

"I'll tell you what Gerald, I'm inclined to think it stands for Jefferson Davis," Cal said.

"The President of the Confederate States?" Ashley asked.

"I'm impressed again, Ashley," Gerald said and smiled.

"I happen to have a particular interest in American wars, Brugge," she replied.

"We can tell you in that bar it sure felt like we were in the antebellum South," Thomas said and Fred nodded.

Ashley also mentioned Sophia said her father-in-law had some diarrhea around the time he sold that litter, but it was not bad enough to see a doctor.

"Interesting. I wonder if he got a little dose of whatever those pigs had that he sold to our patients," Gerald added.

"That's what Sophia thought too," Ashley said.

JUNE 14, 2021, 8:01 A.M.
National Health Center, Respiratory Unit, Doctor's Lounge

Gerald was tapping Jack Durante's number on his cell phone screen. He could not wait to update him.

"Jack, it's Gerald Brugge. Do you have a minute? I have news," he got out in one breath when the CDB epidemiologist answered.

"Gerry, I was getting ready to call you."

"You first, Jack," Gerald said only to be polite.

"We've had 25 more cases reported since we last spoke."

"About a month ago, right?"

"Yes."

"So that's about six new ones a week?"

"Reported ones, anyway," Jack said.

"Are there any hospitalized ones, Jack?"

"A few here in Atlanta. That's why I was calling you. Ready to take them?"

"Believe it or not, Jack, not right now. I think we found the source."

"You're kidding me," Jack said.

"All of our patients here at NHC with this disease have some affiliation with a pig farm. They either bought some pigs there or have some type of personal relationship with the buyers."

"Where's the farm, Gerald?"

"In North Carolina. Clinton."

"Fantastic. How did you learn all of this?"

"I knew we needed nurses to do it, but we could not keep the ones we had originally. These patients are challenging, to say the least. So we hired some AIDS nurses in D.C. who we recruited from the Quilt exhibit. Shift after shift they got what we needed."

"Impressive. I'm assuming these pigs were sick."

"It sure seems to be that way."

"You know, Gerry, it's difficult for humans to contract pig viruses. What did these people do, drink their blood?"

"More like smeared it on. There seems to have been some mucous membrane exposure."

"Damn. I'm going to need veterinarian expertise so we know what we even need to test for."

Then, Jack Durante asked Gerald Brugge for a list of all the symptoms and diseases the NHC patients have experienced over the past month.

After Gerald finished telling him about the high fevers and the *Mycoplasma* pneumonias, and the profound diarrhea and the purple lesions always appearing in conjunction with kidney failure and the secondary *PCP* pneumonias not responding to Pentamidine or Bactrim resulting in ventilation and one death already, and the strong possibility of another one soon, Jack said,

"How interesting. An immune deficiency certainly seems to be in the mix. I'll give my contact in Iowa, at the university, all this information, Gerry, and see what she thinks. We'll find the culprit. So, where's my team headed to exactly in Clinton, N.C.?"

"Porky's Farm. One Tucker Abbott runs it. One of our AIDS nurses working with us now is his daughter-in-law. She prepared him last night for a public health visit."

"It doesn't get any easier than this, Gerald. Your team has practically done our work for us. Thank you."

"No, thank you, Jack. Will you send me some of the samples you collect?"

"Of course. Once we've found the little bug, I will ship them your way. I'm hoping to know tonight after our field trip to Clinton. Will you be on duty, Gerry? It'll probably be late."

"I'm not coming off duty until we know what this is and we develop the vaccine," Gerald said.

JUNE 14, 2021, 11:00 P.M.
National Health Center, Respiratory Unit

Dr. Gerald Brugge was standing with two medical residents, finishing up their Infectious Diseases rotation, in George Johnson's room. Charlie Brown had just called a Code Blue because the patient's heart had stopped beating.

Gerald stepped back to allow the female and male doctors run this emergency. Charlie pumped on the patient's chest with one hand and administered the IV epinephrine the female doctor had just ordered with his other hand, like a dancer in sync with the rhythm of the resuscitation, while the respiratory therapist squeezed the ambu bag, at just the right pause in Charlie's compressions, attached to the endotracheal tube inserted down the patient's throat that was usually connected to the machine.

After two doses of epinephrine, Dr. Brugge read the cardiac monitor. The flat line on the screen had turned into the dangerous pattern that looks like a saw's edge. Gerald took over.

"Let's give him some Amiodarone." Charlie asked the male resident to hand him the syringe of medication from the emergency cart. Then, a few seconds later, the monitor screen looked the same.

"No good," Brugge said. He turned on the machine on top of the emergency cart and instructed the residents to place the pads on the patient's chest so he could deliver the electricity that would jolt Mr. Johnson's heart back into a normal rhythm.

"All clear," Brugge yelled out as the defibrillator machine reached the appropriate charge. Charlie, the respiratory therapist, and the female doctor jumped away from the bed.

The male resident wanted to see where Dr. Brugge placed the paddles to deliver the shock. He did not realize his stethoscope, hanging around his neck, was touching Mr. Johnson's hip as the charge was delivered. The patient's body lifted up off the bed and the young doctor fell to the floor.

"These FNGs," Charlie said as he ran over and started chest compressions on the doctor. He began to cough after only a few seconds of Charlie's intervention.

"What happened?" he asked Charlie.

"All clear means all clear, doc, or you go down while we bring the patient back up," Charlie commanded.

Gerald read the heart monitor and knew it was safe now to stop CPR and leave the patient in Charlie's capable hands. He had to return the call that made his cell phone vibrate in his back pocket during the resuscitation. But first, he needed to explain what just happened to Mrs. Johnson.

He degloved, degowned, and demasked in the ante room and then washed his hands thinking about how many times he had this conversation before stepping out into the hallway.

Mrs. Johnson's face was smeared with tears.

"We saved him, Mrs. Johnson. For now," he told her.

"Praise the Lord. What happened to my Georgie, Dr. Brugge?"

"His heart is starting to shut down. All those fluids are building up. The dialysis is not working the way it has been, Mrs. Johnson, and the pneumonia is clogging up his lungs, making his heart work harder and harder."

"Is he going to live, doctor?"

Gerald learned, back in the old days, to be honest at this point even though it hurt the loved ones to hear the end was so near, but it usually saved them from the sucker punch of Death's next knock.

"For a little while, Mrs. Johnson. Perhaps a few days, maybe only one. If anyone wants to say goodbye to your husband, now is the time. I am very sorry."

"Thank you, doctor," Mrs. Johnson said and buried her face in her hands.

JUNE 14, 2021, 11:45 P.M.
National Health Center, Respiratory Unit, Doctor's Lounge

Dr. Jack Durante answered his cell phone, a number he only gave to a few doctors out in the field.

"Hi, Jack."

"We got it, Gerry."

Durante began with the conversation he had with the Iowa veterinarian expert this morning after he had gotten off the phone with Gerald. Jack told Dr. Lisa Miller all about the diseases in Gerald's NHC patients, asking her if she has seen anything similar in pigs.

"Are you kidding me, Jack? This sounds like classic Porcine Circovirus. We've just never seen it in humans before. Fascinating," she said.

Then Dr. Miller explained to the CDB expert that when the virus initially infects pigs it overstimulates their immune systems, which in turn attacks the pigs' own bodies. Some pigs develop purple lesions from inflamed blood vessels and skin breaking down, and kidney disease leading to failure. Other pigs develop pneumonia, usually *Mycoplasma*.

"Unreal," Gerald said as Jack repeated these details. "That's our patient population."

"I told Lisa that. Then I told her about some of the *PCP* pneumonias you've seen in your sicker patients and she wasn't surprised at all. Pigs who live with this Porcine Circovirus, or PCV, for a while develop white blood cell depletion leading to a substantial immune suppression prior to death."

"Like HIV acts, in a way," Gerald said. "That's why we're seeing the *PCP*."

"That seems to be right," Jack said.

"So how was the trip to Porky's Farm, Jack?"

"One nice farmer, he really was, Gerry. He let us test him, some of his pigs, and the soil."

Tucker Abbott told the CDB doctor about the litter he sold last October being less active than usual. He told Jack he remembered it well because the men who bought the piglets wore white hoods.

"I couldn't believe what he was telling me. Honestly, Gerald, I did not realize the KKK was even active today."

"Me, neither, Jack, until I heard the subject come up over and over again with our patients."

"I had to call Lisa again at that point to ask her what other information would be helpful," Jack said.

The vet told the epidemiologist to ask the farmer if he remembered any other sick pig litters around that time, and if by chance the farmer kept records of the lot numbers from vaccines he had given. "Many farmers do," she said.

Tucker told Jack there were "no other less than hardy litters before or since that one." And lucky for them he was a committed pig vaccinator and kept a ledger filled with all the vaccines he gave his pigs over the past ten years, including the sick litter's mother last Fall.

Tucker preferred to vaccinate the pregnant ones instead of all the little babes. "Just easier," he told Jack.

"Lisa Miller called me later on to tell me Farmer Abbott's PCV vaccine lot numbers, given to the mother of the sick litter, had matched some other ineffective vaccines made during the winter of 2020.

"Lisa said there had been some case reports involving vaccinated pigs who had died from this virus last fall."

"I wonder what caused the bad vaccines, Jack? Was it something in the manufacturing environment?" Gerald asked.

"It seems to be, if you allow the first stage of vaccine production to be considered a part of that environment."

Lisa Miller had explained to Jack how fertilized hen eggs were still used to grow the Porcine Circovirus, and then the viral protein was extracted to make the vaccine. But if the hens are stressed, say, from warmer than usual weather, which happened last winter in the Midwestern U.S.A, the viral protein does not reproduce properly in the hen eggs and the vaccine is much, much weaker.

"Global warming at its best, Jack," Gerald responded.

"Indeed, it is," Jack said.

"So did Mr. Abbott have antibodies in his blood to this PCV, Jack?"

"He sure did. And so did the pigs we tested who were not even vaccinated yet. The soil samples were positive, too. Lisa said it is not unusual for most farms to have positive pigs before vaccination and the virus can live in the soil for a long time. She said many pigs carry the virus but never get sick."

"Like Tucker Abbott," Gerald said and also thought about Betty Ann Williams' husband.

"Well, Farmer Abbott had been sick with diarrhea for about six to eight weeks. He told me, but that was about it. Not enough to land him in the hospital or even see a doctor," Jack said.

"Were you able to send me some specimens, Jack?"

"Sure was. They will be there tomorrow morning. A few vials of Abbott's blood and some pig antibody tests. Lisa arranged for my team to pick up some of these tests at a veterinary college not far from Porky's Farm."

"I collect blood, Jack, on all my patients here at NHC. I developed a consent form decades ago asking for permission to test the blood on any patient admitted for known and unknown viruses, bacteria, any pathogen really. You would be amazed how many patients we had back in the late 1970s who had positive HIV tests when we finally developed the antibody test in the mid-80s."

"I bet. Well, old friend, you have some long hours ahead of you."

"Me and the vaccine team. Oh, one more thing, Jack. Can you ask Dr. Miller if this PCV vaccine works in pigs who are already sick? I'm thinking the vaccine we develop might help my patients from getting any sicker, and really I'm hoping it will make them better."

"I'll be in touch soon, Gerry."

June 15, 2021, 10:00 P.M.
National Health Center, Virology Department

"I think we have it, ladies and gentlemen," Gerald said, holding up a small vial of the vaccine.

"If only HIV could have been so easy," one of the male scientists said.

"Well, we never got it before it mutated, did we? And we did not isolate the virus in 1981 when patients started getting sick. We got this little circovirus pretty darn pure, early in the game." Gerald said.

"Only because the Vice President's son got sick," a female scientist commented.

"True. But we took advantage of that, and we have been studying this small group of patients with the symptoms of this new syndrome. And because of that it looks like we might be preventing another viral catastrophe," Gerald said.

Jack Durante had let Gerald know the good news from the vet expert in Iowa a few hours before the lab produced this first circovirus vaccine for humans. Pigs who have been sick with PCV disease indeed can improve if they are vaccinated. The antibodies produced in their bodies after vaccination provide some protection against further cellular damage from the virus.

"Let's go home and get some sleep, people," Gerald instructed the scientists. "No more death with this gold right here."

JUNE 15, 2021, 3:04 P.M.
National Health Center, Respiratory Unit

The day hospitalist, Dr. Richards, dealt with George Johnson's demise while Dr. Brugge developed the vaccine with his team down in the lab. Sharon, the nurse who had floated to this unit today from the medical ICU, called a Code Blue just a few minutes ago when the patient's heart stopped beating again.

Mrs. Johnson could not bring herself to sign the Do Not Resuscitate Order Nurse Charlie Brown tried to talk to her about last night after the patient's first Code. If she had signed the document, the medical team would have had permission to not pump on the patient's chest, not give medications to stimulate his worn-out heart, and not shock him one last time.

Sharon had asked Mrs. Johnson to wait outside in the hallway while the team attempted the futile rescue. Sharon began pumping again on the patient's chest after injecting one dose of epinephrine and then said, "I don't think all the drugs in the world, Dr. Richards, will get Mr. Johnson dancing again."

"Agreed," the doctor said. "Time 1504."

After the doctor told Mrs. Johnson about her husband's death, he called Gerald Brugge with the news.

Mrs. Johnson cried and cried in the hallway sitting in the linen covered chair Sharon found for her in the visitor's lounge.

"I'm right glad, nurse, Dr. Brugge told me how sick my Georgie was last night," she said with drier eyes.

"I am so sorry, Mrs. Johnson," Sharon said, rubbing her shoulder.

"I only wish the good Lord would've brought our daughter up here to us, to say goodbye to her daddy," she said and the tears began again.

Sharon stayed with Mrs. Johnson for a few more minutes, but then returned to the deceased patient's room to prepare the body for the morgue.

Five minutes later, Nurse Dan Napolina came out of Betty Ann Williams' room and saw Mrs. Johnson sitting in the chair staring straight ahead with a blank look.

"Mrs. J., you alright?" Dan said when he reached her.

"Oh, Danny, my Georgie's gone for good now. God Almighty came to get him."

"I heard, Mrs. J., and I'm really sorry for sure. I guess your daughter didn't make it up here in time."

"She never tried. She wouldn't even talk to him when I called her and told her how sick he was. That was early this morning.

"I held the phone up to my Georgie's ear. Told him it was

Cheryl Lynn. He opened his eyes real wide-like then. I could tell he was happy, but she wouldn't say a word to him.

"Then I took the phone and raised my voice to her. I told her she is one ungrateful child. 'Everything your daddy done for you. Almighty God ain't ever gonna forgive you.'

"Then she said to me, Danny, her own mother who brought her into this world nearly forty years ago. She said, 'Mother, I think you got that all wrong. The good Lord ain't ever gonna forgive Daddy for what he's done to Black folks all his life nor you for lett'n him do it.'"

"That's rough, Mrs. J," Dan said.

"Now I'm all alone in this big world, Danny. Lost my husband's good lov'n and friendship and my only child too."

"You work on repairing things with her, you know, Mrs. J. You have a grandson. And remember, you never wore a hood or played around with pig's blood. Right?"

"My heavens, no."

"Tell your daughter you couldn't help but love your Georgie and you never meant any harm to her or your grandson."

"Thank you, Danny."

"Sure thing. So, look, I need to ask you if you'd let us draw a tube of blood from your arm before you head back home. NHC has a car for you, don't they?"

"Deed they do. And a hearse for my Georgie. But why do you want my blood?"

"Dr. Brugge thought it might be a good idea to see if you have the virus too that made Mr. J. so sick," Dan explained.

"Was it from that pig?"

"The good doc thinks so," Dan said and then shared the information Dr. Brugge gave the staff about the pig virus anti-bodies the CDB found in the farmer's blood where her husband and his friends bought the pigs.

"I hope I don't ever get sick like Georgie, if I do have that virus," she said.

"Slim chance of that happening, Mrs. J. You haven't been sick this whole time. Anyway, Dr. Brugge is working on a vaccine as we speak."

"Thank you for everything, Danny," Mrs. Johnson said and gave him a nice, long hug.

June 16, 2021, 7:00 A.M.
National Health Center, Respiratory Unit

Gerald was only able to sleep last night because he skipped a whole day's rest working in the lab. He wanted to talk with Reba Smith before she was discharged.

He washed his hands in the anteroom and knocked on her door.

"Good Morning, Ms. Reba. We are quite happy you are going home to Alabama," he said.

"I thanks you, doctor, for all your real good care."

"Not good enough, though. I am still so sorry about your husband."

"I knows that. You and all them nurses sure did try. It just seems strange going on home without my Sam."

"We found the cause, Ms. Reba, of your husband's sickness," Gerald said.

"Well, Lordy be. Let's hear it!"

"Human Porcine Circovirus or HPCV."

"My Sam done and got it from that pig, didn't he?" she asked.

"It seems so. His blood had antibodies to the pig virus we found on that farm in North Carolina where he bought the pigs."

"Do you have a treatment for it yet?" Mrs. Smith asked.

"We just developed a vaccine. We're going to give some today," Dr. Brugge explained.

"Do I needs to have it?"

"Well, your blood showed antibodies to the pig virus also."

"So I got it from my Sam?"

"It appears to be unless you had anything to do with that sick pig."

"No, Dr. Brugge. I just looks on it in our pen and tells my Sam it didn't seem right. Do you think Sam gave it to me through some lov'n?" Reba Smith asked.

"I think so."

"So, do I needs that vaccine you made up?"

"Not now. You've recovered, Ms. Reba. If you get sick again, we might give it to you."

"I sure am glad my daughter told me to tell my nurses all about my Sam and those other men and the pig's blood. Deed, it was right embarrassing, though."

"I imagine it was, Mrs. Smith, but it helped us find the virus, and now I'm hoping the cure. Have a safe trip home."

"I thanks you, doctor."

JUNE 16, 2021, 7:30 A.M.
National Health Center, Respiratory Unit, Staff Lounge

Gerald told the nurses at the end of their report now about getting ready to consent the three remaining patients to the clinical trial he just developed for the vaccine. And he told them he usually administers the vaccines on study.

"Sounds good, doc," Dan said. "Just tell us what to look out for today besides localized reactions like we would see with any vaccine."

"And maybe some low-grade temps and chills," Bridgette said even though she was going off duty.

"And perhaps a cytokine release syndrome when the patient starts producing antibodies later in the day," Thomas added.

"Oh, yes, like the cellular treatments for cancer can now cause. Thanks, Thomas. If any of the patients have a particularly strong immune response that could happen."

"I've only read about that syndrome but haven't really seen it," Dan said and Bridgette agreed.

"I am only familiar with it because some of my clinic patients back in Phili have had T cell therapies for some pretty bad herpes infections and experienced it," Thomas said.

"Interesting, Thomas. I've read about some of those trial results," Gerald said and then changed the subject.

"Well, nurses, it looks like your time is short here now."

They smiled.

"All of you have been pure magic for the NHC. I hope you will be in town a few more days so we really can show our appreciation to all of you on Friday night," Gerald said.

"Sure thing, doc. I spoke with Ashley earlier today and she thought the NHC would only need us for a few more shifts anyway since not many patients are left. Plus, she said she hired some new nurses just for this unit," Dan said.

"That's right. Now, I better get busy with my Salk work," the doctor smiled and headed to the lab to get the vaccines.

June 16, 2021, 8:30 A.M.
National Health Center, Respiratory Unit

Gerald went to Betty Ann Williams' room first because he thought he might still be able to save her kidneys from dialysis.

He washed his hands, gowned, and gloved before knocking on her door.

"How are you today, Mrs. Williams?"

"Nice to see you, Dr. Brugge. Shouldn't you be home by now?"

"Usually I am," Gerald said and then explained what they now knew about the cause of this disease, and told her she had been infected with the virus because she had antibodies in her blood.

"You say it's from a pig. Like that sick little one Burt brought on home last fall?"

"I believe so, Mrs. Williams. Did you help your husband care for that pig?"

"No, doctor."

"Did you eat the pig?"

"Heavens no! Burt bought it for the albino children's Christmas dinner, but that pig looked right ill and never made it to the children's plates."

Gerald then told Mrs. Williams she would be the very first person to receive the vaccine, if she gave permission.

"Will it make my kidneys work on their own again without all this medication?" she asked pointing to the IV bag filled with Dopamine.

"We hope," Gerald said.

"Will it make these lesions go away, right quick?"

"We hope so."

The patient agreed to sign the consent form, but first Gerald asked her if she had any more questions.

"Just one, Dr. Brugge. How did I get this virus if I didn't have anything to do with that little sick pig no how?"

"Your husband did though, right? I mean he touched it and fed it."

"Yes, doctor. And he told me he ended up killing it too," she said.

"I'd like to test your husband's blood, for the antibodies to the pig virus. I suspect he has it."

"Why isn't he sick then, doctor?"

"Not everyone gets sick."

"The virus comes from marital relations, Dr. Brugge?"

"Well, it comes from pigs and it looks like it can be passed along through sex," he explained.

"I have some praying to do for some people, I believe," she said.

Gerald did not respond to her comment and asked her to sign the consent form now. Then he gave her the vaccine in her arm.

"I will call your husband, Mrs. Williams, and ask him to have his blood drawn at a local hospital in Atlanta."

"He'll do it. I know my Burt. Thank you, doctor."

"Thank you, Mrs. Williams."

JUNE 16, 2021, 2021, 9:15 A.M.
National Health Center, Respiratory Unit

James Wilson had just returned from dialysis so Gerald gowned and gloved up and then knocked on his door.

"Come on in, whoever you are. I'll take what I can get at this point. The color don't matter none."

"Hello, Mr. Wilson," Gerald entered his room and thought, how on earth have the nurses taken care of this man?

"Well, hello, Dr. Brugge. You're a mighty white sight for sore eyes. Now tell me then, are my kidneys going to get better? I got a restaurant that needs tending to. My poor Emma can't do it on her own forever."

"I have some good news. We found the cause of your disease," Gerald said.

"Great. You can move on to curing it then."

"Well, we just developed the vaccine."

"Sign me up, doctor."

Gerald explained to Mr. Wilson, if he agreed to the vaccine, he would be watched with the other two patients for any bad side effects for at least another week.

"Do you think it's going to work?"

"We sure hope so."

"How did I get this thing, Dr. Brugge?"

"Your disease, the virus you have, comes from a pig," Brugge said and then explained the tracing of the sick litter back to a North Carolina farm.

"Was it Porky's there in Clinton?" Mr. Wilson asked.

"As a matter of fact, it was. You've heard of the farm?"

"Heard of it, hell, I've been there. Last Halloween time. Bought two pigs myself. Small ones."

"Did you eat any of the pig meat?" Gerald asked and could see James Wilson get a little pale.

"Never did take a bite," Mr. Wilson said.

"Did you buy the pigs to cook in your restaurant?"

"Nope. Bought 'em for our charity. Pigs got real sick though and never made it onto their table."

"Albino children, right?" Brugge asked.

"How'd you know, doc?"

"Lucky guess," Gerald said and gave him the vaccine after he signed the consent form.

June 16, 2021, 10:00 A.M.
National Health Center, Respiratory Unit

Gerald was standing in Ronnie Lynch's anteroom now washing his hands. As he put on his gown and gloves, he thought about how this young man's kidneys suffered so much damage.

The best case scenario for him would be continued dialysis until a kidney match for transplant was found.

But without the vaccine, or if the vaccine did not work, Gerald knew Ronnie would not even make it to transplant.

"Hello, Ronnie," Gerald said after he knocked and then entered the room of the bloated boy too weak to stand on his own after the dialysis he had earlier this morning.

"Ronnie, I do have some good news," Gerald said.

"I'm happy to hear any news, Dr. Brugge. I can't believe I've been here a month. My last exam and Georgetown seem years away."

"I bet they do, Ronnie. We found the cause of your disease."

"What is it?"

"A virus."

"HIV?"

"No, remember you've been tested for that."

"I might not have converted yet."

"We tested your blood again last week. Are you that worried about having it?"

"I am, doctor."

"Did you have a risky encounter?"

"Yes."

"When, approximately?"

"Over my Spring break, back in March."

Gerald explained to Ronnie he most likely would have

seroconverted to HIV by now, but he should be tested every month until September.

"If it's not HIV, *yet*, what is it, doctor?"

"It's a pig virus. Porcine Circovirus, it's called in pigs. We've found it jumped from pigs to humans."

"I don't even eat pork. And it's not like I have a lot of exposure to farm animals in Georgetown," Ronnie said.

"I know but you could have contracted it during sex."

Ronnie started to cry. "I knew I should not have gone to that bar in Atlanta."

"It's OK, Ronnie."

"I'm fine, Dr. Brugge. Sorry I got soft. So, tell me what's the good news or was that it?"

Gerald was relieved to be able to jump into his vaccine trial explanation and leave behind a more detailed conversation about Ronnie Lynch's Atlanta experience.

"Do you think it will work?"

"We hope so. There's a good chance it will help stop any further damage to your body, especially your kidneys."

"Will these ugly purple things go away?" Ronnie asked as he lifted his gown.

"We'll see."

"Will I get off dialysis?"

"We'll see, Ronnie," Gerald said and gave the third HPCV vaccine after the young man signed the consent.

June 16, 2021, 7:15 P.M.
National Health Center, Respiratory Unit, Staff Lounge

"I don't know what the hell's going on out there but it's starting to fuckin' feel like 1987," Dan Napolina said as he entered the lounge, late for report, with the night shift waiting along with Ashley Smith. "Pardon my mouth," Dan added.

Even though the vaccine patients sailed through the day with the worst reaction being Betty Ann Williams' low-grade temperature of 100.4, the last two hours brought in a storm of unexpected admissions from the ER.

Earlier, Ashley had asked to speak with the ER medical director when an ER nurse called Dan around 4:30 P.M. trying to give report on a new patient with purple lesions.

"Dr. Brugge did not want any more patients with HPCV illnesses until the safety of the vaccines is established in our patients, Doug," Ashley told the director.

"I don't know what you're talking about, Ashley, but it doesn't matter. This guy we'd like to send up, Randy Humboldt, has been faithfully taking PrEP for years now, but it's no longer covered," he said.

"OK, Doug, now I don't know what you're talking about."

"Pre-exposure prophylaxis. The pills that prevent HIV transmission," he told her.

"This patient has HIV?" Ashley asked.

"No, Ashley, this patient has full blown AIDS. He became HIV positive a few months ago, he tells us, because he could not afford the meds. And he's a 31-year-old D.C. attorney. Now he has KS everywhere, below his neck, that is, but primarily in his lungs. At least that's what the scans show."

"You better send him up, Doug. Thanks."

Ashley helped Dan with the computer part of the admission. Even though Betty Ann Williams' hourly assessments were less intense, Dan needed to focus on the direct care required for Mr. Humboldt.

Blood needed to be drawn, urine and sputum needed to be collected, chemotherapy orders needed to be checked for dosing before it was prepared by the pharmacy, and vital signs needed to be taken every 30 minutes.

Ashley saved Dan about an hour of work by obtaining the patient's medical, surgical, and medication history, and performing and charting a physical, psychological, and social assessment.

She now told Bridgette, Jack, and Charlie, who she had asked to come in tonight to take care of Betty Ann Williams, "I've never really seen anyone with AIDS before."

"For sure you have not then, Ashley. We've had all the good antiretrovirals since you've been a nurse," Jack said.

"Until now," Bridgette said. "It's inhumane ARVs are no longer covered by insurance. It won't take long, though, for the government to give it back when they start dropping like flies again and hospitals start losing a shit load of money."

"This young man is really sick," Ashley said.

"And it's going to get much worse from here, Ash, and faster than you can ever imagine,' Dan chimed in as he reentered the lounge.

"I felt terrible I had to page Brugge a few hours ago. I held off after Mr. Humboldt was admitted, but then Ms. Vasquez came up from the ER not long after him."

"Another one?" Bridgette commented.

"Yes, it's unreal really. Thomas will give you report on her. I also completed her admission. She has *PCP*. She told me the last time she had this pneumonia was in 1997, right before she went on the medications. She said they saved her life. Obviously, they did."

"Let me guess then, Ashley, she cannot afford them now," Jack said.

"That's right. She has been taking the same combo pill since 2006 and it would cost her $20,000 per month without insurance. How outrageous is that!" Ashly finished.

Now she remembered the conversation she had with Gerald at *The Holocaust Museum*. So, this is what can happen, she thought.

After Charlie received report from Dan on Mrs. Williams, he told Bridgette and Jack he would help out with their patients tonight. He could see Mrs. Williams required less time because the nurses had been tapering down the Dopamine dose every two hours, ever since her kidneys started to produce more urine throughout the day.

Charlie remembered how sick AIDS patients got before the antiretroviral revolution. He told them he would watch over James Wilson while Jack administered the chemotherapy for the Kaposi's Sarcoma patient and check in on Ronnie Lynch while Bridgette gave the *PCP* patient IV antibiotics, respiratory treatments, and performed vital signs every fifteen minutes.

"We owe you a bit of a wee drink then, Charlie," Jack said.

"More like a big one, or two," Bridgette said.

"Sounds good. I'm going in," Charlie said and darted out to the floor to take care of patients.

JUNE 16, 2021, 8:15 P.M.
National Health Center, Nursing Supervisor's Office

Ashley sat down in her chair and sighed. She at least took some solace in knowing she still had her AIDS nurses for tomorrow's day and night shifts, more agency nurses were coming who took one month contracts, and two new permanent nurses were hired just for her respiratory unit.

And she would feel really satisfied right now, if the phone calls she was about to make turned out the way she was hoping.

"Oh, hello, Ashley," Linda Washington picked up the phone in her hotel room.

"Tomorrow? I will be there at 0650."

"Thank you so much, Linda."

June 16, 2021, 8:30 P.M.
Crystal Nightingale Hotel

Linda knew Cal would be working tomorrow so she called to let her know Ashley had just asked her to work as a preceptor, one on one, with a new nurse from Seattle.

"Did we get more sick ones?" Cal asked.

"Yes, Cal, but our kind of sick," Linda said.

"It's happening already. I better call Teddy. See you in the morning, honey," Cal said.

June 16, 2021, 8:35 P.M.
Crystal Nightingale Hotel

Ashley made the next phone call in between the paperwork she was trying to finish up for the night.

"Sura, I hope I am not disturbing you. It's Ashley Smith from NHC."

"Not at all, Ashley. What can I do for you?"

"I need you tomorrow night. I've hired two young nurses, one from Seattle and one from Boston. This might seem like a strange request, and I might be a tad too hopeful about it all, but I thought if these two new nurses could take care of their very first patients with two of the very first AIDS nurses in our country, it would be an invaluable experience for them."

"Well, sure, Ashley. I would be honored. I don't think I can insert an IV after all these years or give medication with enough dexterity or speed."

"Oh, that's not why I want you and Linda. I just need both of you to be you and teach these nurses how to interact with, respond to, and care for AIDS patients."

"I think we might be able to do that better with some actual AIDS patients."

"You can, Sura. Two have just been admitted today."

"I see," Sura said. "I will be there tomorrow night."

June 16, 2021, 10:00 P.M.
Crystal Nightingale Hotel

It took Sura the last hour and a half to explain to Liz why it was a good idea to go into the NHC tomorrow night for just one shift.

"When's the last time you actually cared for an AIDS patient Sura? Twenty years ago?"

"At least. I'm old. Ashley knows that. I don't have to give meds or start IVs. The young nurse will do all that. Ashley needs Linda and me to just be ourselves and show them how to care for someone with AIDS."

"Why can't Sophia do that? She's on tomorrow night, isn't she?"

"Yes, Liz, but there are other patients to care for. Sophia would not have that kind of time to devote for a whole shift."

"I'm worried," Liz said.

"That it will hurt me?" Sura said.

"Yes, Sura. You've suffered a lot."

"Well, this shift will be more about passing a torch."

"Not if it burns you, Sura."

"I need to call Sophia, Liz."

PART 4

ONE MORE SHIFT

J<small>UNE</small> 17, 2021, 7:45 A.M.
National Health Center, Respiratory Unit

Shift report was over. Linda Washington read through the patient's history on a computer pad in the staff lounge after Bridgette Delaney finished talking about Maria Vasquez's night.

It took all of her shift for Bridgette to get the patient's temperature down to 100 degrees Fahrenheit. At midnight, it was 103. The second dose of antibiotics at 2:00 A.M. helped the fever, but the ice packs Bridgette placed in the patient's armpits and groin area did the trick.

"I went old school," she told them.

"It always worked for me, Bridgette," Linda said.

Linda walked towards Maria Vasquez's room with Ebony Chen, the new day nurse Ashley had hired. Ebony was from Seattle, Washington, but wanted to move east as soon as she graduated from nursing school.

"Do you prefer if I call you Nurse Washington, Mrs. or Ms. Washington, or Linda?" Ebony asked in the hallway.

"Do you prefer if I call you Nurse Chen, Ms. Chen, or Ebony?" Linda asked in turn.

"I think for my first day on duty I would like to be called Nurse Chen. Nursing school was hard and I'd like to feel the success of completing it."

"Well you should, Nurse Chen. But your real success as a nurse begins today as you start to figure out how to make patients feel the best they can while providing medical care.

"There's no handbook, no textbook, and no right way to do that," Linda explained.

"No one ever taught me that in nursing school, Nurse Washington."

"Please call me Linda. Now, do you have any questions about this patient before we go in?" Linda asked because she knew Ebony had also read the patient's chart during report.

"How can we make it so Ms. Vasquez doesn't get sick like this again?"

"Great question, Nurse Chen. We have returned to a bad time. I don't know how much you know about the dark years before the ARV revolution in the mid-1990s. The virus circulated unchecked and attacked the immune system which led to all types of crazy infections no one ever heard about before," Linda said.

"You mean like PML?" Ebony asked.

"Indeed. How do you know about Progressive Multifocal Leukoencephalopathy?"

"My father died from it last year."

"Was he receiving immunotherapy for cancer or MS or arthritis?" Linda asked knowing that treatment can cause, in rare cases, this horrible brain disease.

"No. He stopped taking his HIV meds when his insurance stopped covering it."

"No one should ever have to see that infection, certainly not in one's own father," Linda said.

"It's why I chose this hospital and unit, to be involved with treating infectious diseases. I figured my dad was not the only one out there dying from AIDS. I don't want anyone else to die from it," Ebony said.

"Me neither, Nurse Chen. Let's go in there and see what we can do," Linda said and patted the young nurse's shoulder.

June 17, 2021, 8:00 A.M.
National Health Center, Respiratory Unit

Ebony asked Linda why the room was so dark while they washed their hands in the anteroom. Linda explained the patient's high temperature last night probably caused a headache and some photosensitivity.

"Are we putting on gloves?" Ebony asked as they dried their hands.

"Just a mask for now. Keep some gloves in your pocket in case we encounter any fluids. But there's no need for them if we don't. Always wash your hands before you touch any patients and after, too. The mask we will need until her third sputum specimen comes back negative for TB," Linda explained.

Linda knocked on Maria Vasquez's door. Some light followed her and Ebony into the room.

"Don't turn them lights on!" the patient shouted.

"No problem, Ms. Vasquez. May I open the blinds just a little bit so we can see each other?" Linda asked.

"Alright," the patient huffed.

After Linda turned the blades of the blinds, just enough, she said, "Ms. Vasquez, are you feeling any better since last night? We know you had one heck of a temperature."

"Damn straight I did. Felt like my head was going to pop off. I cursed that night nurse when she placed those ice bags on me, but after fifteen minutes I couldn't thank her enough."

"May we take your temperature now?" Linda asked.

The patient nodded her head yes. The electronic thermometer read 99.4 when it beeped.

"Very nice, Ms. Vasquez. May we listen to your lungs?" Linda asked.

The patient said yes.

"What do you hear, Nurse Chen?" Linda asked after she pulled her stethoscope away from the patient.

"It sounds like rales in the bases," Ebony said as she moved the diaphragm on her instrument to the upper lobes of the patient's lungs next. "Clear here."

"Very good," Linda said.

"What do you think, nurses?" the patient asked.

"You still have some fluid in there. It seems like the antibiotics are working though. By the way, Ms. Vasquez, I am Linda and this is Nurse Ebony Chen. We will be your nurses until the evening."

"Why the two of you? You look a little too old and you look a little too young," Ms. Vasquez said moving her eyes from Linda to Ebony.

"Well, I guess we'll come out just right in the middle then," Linda said with a smile. "I am orienting Nurse Chen today."

"What do you know about my disease, a disease that went away a long time ago. At least, it should have."

"I worked in San Francisco," Linda said.

"Back then, nurse?" the patient asked.

"Please call me Linda. Yes, back then. I moved there in '83, from Texas."

"You worked with us?" the patient asked.

"Yes, on the first AIDS Unit."

"Damn."

"Yes, Ms. Vasquez."

"You call me Maria."

"I read in your chart, Maria, that you are from New York City," Linda said.

"I am."

"How long have you lived in D.C.?"

"I can't afford to live in the District, as they say down here. I live in Silver Spring, Md., not too far away. I came down here after I got clean.

"All that modeling I did in the city back then got me in a whole lot of trouble. Sure was fun while it lasted, though," Maria said with a smile.

Linda stood there listening to this patient but Iris Ortega was the face she saw now, her first female AIDS patient at Bay City General. Linda stopped herself from drifting back.

She listened to Maria Vasquez tell Ebony about the model-ing, her husband who started off as her agent, all the cocaine, then the heroin, then the needles, then the HIV, and then her husband's death.

Ebony responded, "My father was from Chinatown in New York. It sounds like you might have hung out in the same clubs back then. He used to tell me and my mom all about the Studio."

"Those were the days, baby. The days. Muchá diversion, lots of fun."

Linda said, "I'm beginning to regret not making it to that club. One of the East Coast AIDS nurses with us now told me all about it too."

"Where did she work, Linda?" Maria asked.

"Upper East Side Medical Center. Did you ever go there, Maria?"

"No way. Too far uptown for me. I always ended up at Village Community."

"We have some of those nurses with us now, too," Linda said.

"I know. My night nurse, Bridgette, remembered me. I did not remember her. I was too fucked up on dope and toxoplasmosis back then, most of the time anyway."

Linda explained this parasitic infection to Ebony that often went to the brains of AIDS patients. She also explained how many of her patients were terrified of cats because their litter boxes could harbor the bug.

"You know, that might be why my dad never let me have a cat. He would always say, 'puppies OK. Cats stay away,'" Ebony said to Linda and the patient.

"What did your dad do in New York, Nurse Chen?" the patient asked her.

"Please call me Ebony, Ms. Vasquez. He was an interior designer, really a carpenter. He built everything he designed. He told me and my mom he had clients up and down Madison and Park Avenues."

"That's how he got into the Studio," the patient said.

"I guess so. He used to say he should have shot for lower stars because then he wouldn't have gotten such a taste for the high life," Ebony said.

"You said you're from Seattle, Ebony?" the patient asked.

"I am, Ms. Vasquez."

"Call me Maria. Is that where your mom is from, too?" the patient asked.

"She is. They met right after he got out of rehab. There's a really good center there. That was in 1996. He tested positive for HIV but he got on the meds."

"He was lucky, Ebony. I was positive in 1990 and got sick quite a few times before the good combos came out," Maria said.

"You're right. My dad was lucky. I, really we, me and my mom, never knew what AIDS looked like because he was always so healthy. My mom never got it and then I was born. I never got it either."

"See that's the kinda good stuff that happened with HAART. It gave us all regular lives again, with side effects. But that was alright. That's why when I got clean I went to college. Managed to save some of my modeling money.

"I studied public policy and became a lobbyist right here in D.C. Fought hard for those drugs to be covered by insurances with affordable copays. But not anymore."

Maria Vasquez continued. "What we have now in this country is a virtual concentration camp created by that president of ours and his government. All the virus carriers, all the gays, trans, all the women, all of us people of color who don't fit into Rumpel's white, heterosexual male, and Christian world, or what he claims is Christian, are suffering or dying now from neglect of our needs and civil rights."

"You are so right, Maria," Linda spoke now while encouraging Ebony to hang the antibiotic. "You will learn how to do both," she told Ebony. "It's tricky at first because you want to stop and only listen to the patient or just focus on giving the med. With experience, you will be able to do both at the same time, Ebony."

Linda turned to the patient. "I don't know about you, Maria, but I never thought I'd see the '80s again."

"It's back, baby. Who could've ever imagined. And it's much worse," Maria said. "Now, thank you nurses for your care but you have truly tired me out. I'll see you in a few." She pulled the covers over her head.

Linda closed the blinds and said, "We'll be back later, Maria. Call if you need anything."

Linda and Ebony took off their masks and washed their hands in the anteroom. "You're going to be a good nurse, Nurse Chen. You share yourself. That's what makes them trust you, makes them feel comfortable. Just be careful and don't share too much or you'll get real hurt, real fast."

Linda led Ebony into the hallway.

June 17, 2021, 8:30 A.M.
National Health Center, Respiratory Unit

Cal was relieved to get out of James Wilson's room. The patient did not have dialysis today, and probably would not need it tomorrow. He felt better and that meant more talking.

Cal could not get the conversation out of her head, standing in the hallway outside of Randy Humboldt's room.

"You mean to tell me, a woman like yourself who seems alright to me, in spite of forgetting your position in this world, ain't been down home to Mississippi in how long?"

"More than two decades, going on three," Cal said.

"On account of livin' all the way out there in Queersville?" Mr. Wilson asked after Cal added she lived in San Francisco.

"On account of Southerners like you who say the ugliest of things about other people and places, Mr. Wilson."

"Hmmm," he said and not another word while Cal gave him his medications.

Cal thought now, it might be Mr. Wilson kept his mouth shut because he just might have realized, for a minute, how nasty he was. Wishful thinking, 'deed.

She washed her hands in the anteroom looking through the glass part of the door at the young man sleeping in the bed.

The last time Stephen visited Cal she was looking at Betty Ann Williams' purple lesions. The young man in this room had the real deal though. For this moment, Cal was safe from the encounter with actual KS and AIDS, but not from the past that refused to loosen its grip.

They took care of Stephen De Grasio in 1992. His face had not been spared. Everyone could see how gorgeous Stephen was, had been, if only all of the cancer could be peeled away, especially the crater-sized one in the middle of his forehead hovering over both eyes.

"Achilles turned into a cyclops," Cal told Sophia and the other nurses during report the day Stephen had been admitted to the AIDS Unit at Upper East Side Medical.

Stephen was a fashion photographer. His clients, his models, knew the man's beauty behind the camera surpassed their own. Yet Stephen managed to capture his models' best shots in spite of last minute pimples popping up or an unwanted pound piling on the night before a shoot after indulging in more than one Tic Tac for dinner.

What struck Cal now was how Stephen had remembered every person he ever had sex with, mostly men but there were some women, too. He would say, "Each of them made me who I am. Every one of my marks represents a partner I had."

"Lordy be, Stevie," Cal said back then. "You sure about that?"

"I am, Cali." Stephen called Cal that after Cal shared how he always wanted to be a woman and was going to do it someday soon.

"I wrote down all of their names in this little book right here," Stephen told Cal.

And one morning Cal started to read it. "My heavens, Stevie, there must be thousands in here."

"4,780, to be exact."

"Damn. That's a whole lot of action, sweetie."

"And interaction with other human beings who are now a part of me," Stephen had said.

"I never looked at it like that before," Cal replied.

"My parents sure don't. Or my brothers and sisters. Everyone I've ever loved tells me I have the mark of the devil, the punishment for my sins. But I feel like I'm wearing the mural I've created, my life's work."

Cal could still hear Stephen's exposition, like an artist on opening night.

Cal left Stephen in the anteroom and was getting ready to greet the man in this room as if she had never cared for anyone with AIDS. She would be fresh for Mr. Randy Humboldt.

JUNE 17, 2021, 8:45 A.M.
National Health Center, Respiratory Unit

"Knock, knock, Mr. Humboldt," Cal said, opening the patient's door. "I am Cal Moore, your day nurse today. How are you feeling? I imagine the chemo you received last evening took away some of your appetite and your energy, right quick."

"Good Morning, Cal. Call me Randy. It's too hard to tell. I've been feeling bad baseline for months now," Randy said.

"You can tell me about all that, if you'd like, Randy. Take your time, please. I've got plenty of it for you right now," Cal said.

Randy began by telling Cal about his conversion to HIV when his insurance stopped covering his Pre-exposure Prophylaxis medicine.

"Simply barbaric, it sure is," Cal commented on the loss of coverage, but did not offer any personal information regarding her own HIV positive status or how she had been taking fairly cheap antiretrovirals produced by the pharmaceutical companies not sanctioned by the government.

"You might have some options in the not too distant future, Randy," Cal said knowing her husband and other Right to Live with AIDS activists were working on transporting APIs, active pharmaceutical ingredients, in double and triple combination pills, to the San Francisco company, Sansvir, that had the manufacturing capability to make ARVs from these raw materials.

As Cal understood it, RLA members connected with supply trucks driven by other undercover RLA members, employed by these API companies, headed to government-approved facilities, but funneled enough of the ingredients into the trucks making it to Sansvir's plant.

RLA planned to sell Sansvir's pills as "herbals" online for a low price and hopefully not raise any red flags for government spies looking to squelch the sale of any affordable HIV medication.

"I sure hope so, Cal. I never thought I'd ever have to deal with HIV, let alone AIDS. I only became positive after my wife died."

"From AIDS?"

"No. She committed suicide. I still can't believe she's gone."

"Lordy be, honey. Would you like to share?"

Randy Humboldt went back to his childhood after Cal listened to his lungs and bowels. He tried to talk while Cal examined his mouth for any sores or bleeding and searched for any sign of rash from the chemotherapy on his skin left unmauled by the KS.

"Your face stands in defiance of the cancer," Cal said.

"It's the only free space, Cal. I hope it stays that way."

"It very well might, Randy," Cal said hanging a steroid ordered to help with some of the side effects from chemotherapy. And then she put up a fresh bag of Normal Saline while Randy told her about growing up in Allentown, a city forty miles or so north of Philadelphia, about his traditional German family who had immigrated to the United States after World War I, and about his parents who could understand a lot better than his grandparents his coming out in college in 2008.

"That's right. You were born in 1990. Everyone is so dang young here. I mean the newer nurses, even our supervisor is your age, Randy."

"Forgive me, Cal, but you were young once, too. You still seem young to me."

"I sure don't feel sixty-four. And I know I don't look it," Cal said snapping her fingers up high and then sitting down next to her patient swinging her right leg over her left one.

Randy smiled, almost laughed, and continued to tell Cal about law school in Philadelphia and then his move to D.C. to work for the CLO. That's where he met Lulu, another lawyer a little older than him specializing in LGBT law but in particular transgender cases.

"I have a sister named Lulu down home in Mississippi," Cal said.

"My Lulu was from Alabama, born Louis Lawrence."

"When did she become her true self?" Cal asked.

"Like in 2010, long before we met. After law school but before the bar. Lulu always wanted to take the bar as a woman, wanted to be 'legally blonde.' She sure was."

Cal laughed. "Hot, hot, hot."

"I think I fell in love with her the minute I saw her in the lobby of our law office on K Street. That fuscia Armani suit of hers.

"She was fierce in the courtroom. I used to love to watch her in action.

"'Excuse me, Ma'am,' she began with a boss of a client of hers who was fired for being trans.

'My client, you have said for the record today, and in her employee evaluations, is the best administrative assistant you have ever had. Never missed a day of work, kept you moving from appointment to appointment on time, and handled diffi-cult customers on the phone for you.

'Yet you fired her when someone else in the office told you she was not a *real* woman.

'That's right,' the employer replied under oath.

'Tell me, please, what a real woman is exactly. Someone with children? Do you have children Ms. Appel?' She did not.

'Well, my client adopted a boy when he was only five years old and now he is on scholarship to Harvard.

'Or do we think being a real woman involves how well our suits match our shoes, how coiffed our hair stays throughout the day, or how well our makeup enhances our outfit for daywear and then eveningwear. Because, Ms. Appel, if that is the case, my client has outdone you for sure.'

"The courtroom exploded with laughter. The jury voted in favor of Lulu's client who ended up not returning to that job because she was offered a much better one by one of the jurors after court was adjourned that day."

"Love it, love it, Randy. What on earth happened to her?"

Randy explained when the conversion centers started appearing in 2019, they had been married for two years. Lulu could not win those cases. She tried classifying them as hate centers but the circuit court judges Rumpel appointed only upheld the President's interests.

"Lulu was arrested and forced to go into one of them. She

never hid who she was. The courts declared her an illegal person."

"She was already a woman. Did they think Lulu would go back to being a man mentally, emotionally, physically when she never ever felt like that man?" Cal was getting upset and nervous. She did not want to reveal her own becoming, although Randy had a feeling. That's why he felt so comfortable talking to Cal.

"I appealed and appealed. I got nowhere. They wouldn't even let me visit, see my Lulu behind some glass at least. They were kind enough to call me, though, when they found her hanging from the shower rod in the bathroom."

"My heavens. That poor thing. You poor thing," Cal said.

Randy went onto explain Lulu was HIV positive and on ARVs. He started taking PrEP when they started dating. Randy remained HIV negative until his insurance stopped paying for the meds last year, not long after Lulu died.

Randy was able to pay for his medication out of pocket for a few months but that was about it. He wanted to take the ARVs until he was done trying to "fuck away his pain," as he described it.

But the pain did not go away and the HIV did not stay away. He knew he had the virus when he developed a fever with some flu-like symptoms within a few weeks of his last fling off of PrEP.

"Then the KS came," Randy told Cal. "At first I thought I was just bruising easily. I've never seen KS before."

Cal was flushing Randy's IV line after the steroid finished infusing, thinking how wonderful it must be to live in a world where you did not know what KS looks like.

"And now here I am, Cal. I know I'll die from it if I can't get some medication to halt the virus' replication. This chemotherapy won't do shit for the cancer if the virus is still racing around in my body."

"So true, Randy, but let's see what happens. You are at the National Health Center and the doctor on this unit is one of the original AIDS doctors."

"Wow, Cal, I feel a little better. Thank you."

"You get your rest now. Don't hesitate to ring," Cal said rubbing Randy's back.

Randy smiled for a few seconds while Cal walked out of his room.

JUNE 17, 2021, 1:15 P.M.
National Health Center, Respiratory Unit, Staff Lounge

Linda heard her orientee talking to Margarita with a casual familiarity only experienced in youth.

Iris Ortega was sitting with Linda during this break as if she was returning the favor all these years later. Iris was always alone on the AIDS Unit at Bay City General in 1985, and had felt it since she was the only female patient at that time.

Iris was happy to have the company of the nurses, especially the female ones. She would invite them to sit down, "Háblame," talk to me, she always said.

She did not trust men, period. Her stepfather had made her his little "doll baby," as he called her, carrying her into his bed when her mother worked night shifts as an ICU nurse in L.A. where Iris grew up. She was ten when all of that began.

Linda was thinking about Iris telling the nurses why she never said a word to her mother about her stepfather. She did not want to worry her. Iris knew they were lucky to have made it to Los Angeles from Caborca, a desert region in Mexico almost 500 miles away. Iris was two years old then when she made it across with her mother and Abuela.

Her father was not so lucky. He was caught and they never saw him again. The only memory Iris had of her father was his carrying her around while she held onto the Madre Virgen medal he always wore around his neck. She felt safe then.

Cal walked into the lounge now and smiled as she poured some coffee, noticing Ebony and Margarita talking like they had known each other for years. Cal thought, those were the days feeling like you had so much in common with someone else simply because you were the same age. In another couple of decades, they'll realize how rare it is to find someone who has even walked a few steps down the same path you have.

"Hi honey. You OK?' Cal said to Linda as she stirred her coffee.

Linda just nodded.

"Thinking about someone, Linda? It's hard, hard, hard not to right now. Mine's Stephen from '92. Never saw KS like that before or since, until today," Cal said.

Linda was relieved she did not have to explain to Cal what she was experiencing. And for the first time, after knowing Cal and her husband for years now, she felt like she wanted to share with Cal.

"Iris Ortega. She was so beautiful, a big-time model. Her mother brought her to L.A. from Mexico in the late '50s. Lots of men took advantage of her in some awful ways starting with her stepfather and ending with her agent who got her on the cover of top fashion magazines but the whole time fed her cocaine, then heroin, then both. That was in the late '70s, she told us."

"Terrible, just terrible. Everyone I took care of addicted to speed balling would have sold their souls to the devil just to get that next high," Cal said.

"What's speed balling?" Margarita asked now as she half listened to the older nurses while Ebony told her about where she was from and how she felt fortunate, in terms of her rich cultures, to be Chinese from her father and Black from her mother, but not so much in terms of the U.S. President Rumple wanted these days.

"People who shoot up, or inject, both cocaine and heroin," Cal answered her.

"I guess technically it could be any methamphetamine and opioid," Linda added.

"That doesn't sound good," Margarita said.

"I think that's what my dad did before rehab," Ebony said.

"I'm sure he must've suffered coming off of that stuff," Cal said. Ebony shook her head.

Then Cal said to Linda, "Go on, honey. Sorry to interrupt you."

"When she came to our unit, Iris weighed under 50 lbs. You could still see her beauty, though, if you imagined more layers of muscle and fat applied to her face.

"We always struggled to find a vein on her that had not been used. And we always needed one for antibiotics and fluids. *PCP* pneumonia."

"Challenging, to say the least. We had the no vein crowd back in New York, too," Cal said.

"Iris was one tough cookie. I know Fred must remember her even though he never really got to know her. None of us did, really, but she would not let male nurses do too much with her at all."

"Because of the abuse she had experienced," Cal added.

"Most definitely. She never gave us too many details but you could see, feel really, that big hole in her she just couldn't fill up. She tried to do it with the attention and admiration she got from modeling, and then the drugs that she thought made her feel good but really just dulled her pain."

"That's the way my father saw it, Linda. I think so anyway," Ebony said. "He was in recovery since I was born but he never forgot how using drugs was not about feeling good but about smashing down the bad."

"You're very insightful, Ebony," Cal said.

"We're calling her Nurse Chen today, Cal," Linda added.

"Excuse meeee, Nurse Chen," Cal said with a smile.

"Listening to you nurses, I'm starting to feel like I don't even come close to deserving the title yet," Ebony said.

"I've felt like that ever since I've been working with them over the past few weeks, Ebony, and I've been a nurse for three years," Margarita said. "But I've learned so much from them. I am sorry to see all of you go. There's so much more I need to know."

"There is, Margarita. And you'll learn just what you need to over time with every patient you take care of and from other nurses you work with," Linda said.

"OK now, nurses. Linda, honey, you finish up your story about Iris Ortega," Cal commanded.

Linda told them Iris never did go home. There was no home to return to anyway. All that money she made was gone.

"What made me think about Iris today was Ms. Vasquez telling Nurse Chen and me about how she managed to save some money from her modeling days and get off the drugs and go to college. How sad Iris Ortega could not, did not," Linda explained.

"Oh, that is, Linda. But it really doesn't matter now does it? Ms. Vasquez is headed in the same direction as Ms. Ortega from 1985. Without any ARVs, that is," Cal said.

"Boy, do we need them stat," Linda said.

"'Deed, we do. Did Iris die peacefully, Linda?" Cal asked

and then turned to Ebony and Margarita. "You should know this, girls, nurses, that was the measure of how good our care was back then."

Ebony's eyes widened and she watched Linda as she continued with the story.

"I'll tell you this much, that little woman had enough fire in her, literally, to get everyone's attention before she left this world for good," Linda said.

Iris had developed HIV dementia and most of the time she could not remember her last name or what room she was in. All of that happened about two months after she was admitted.

The nurses usually managed to confiscate her matches and light her cigarettes for her whenever she wanted one. Linda had to explain how back in the 1980s patients were still allowed to smoke in hospitals, not so much in their rooms but in smoking lounges.

"It happened on nights, of course. All the really crazy things usually did," Linda said. "It was a Sunday morning. I know it had to be because I was expecting a quiet shift and Sundays always were. Plus, I remember looking forward to our weekly brunches with entertainment and food provided by one of our local San Francisco caterers.

"But it smelled like something had burnt badly when I got off the elevator. It was still dark outside so it must have been wintertime. The two night nurses looked shell shocked, more so than the usual look of several deaths."

"You mean more than one person can die during the night?" Ebony asked Linda.

Margarita said, "I helped with Sam Smith's body a few weeks ago but he was my first."

"Ebony, sweetie, we sometimes had two or three deaths on one shift back in New York. Those were the good 'ol days," Cal snapped her fingers, but not up high.

Linda went on to tell them the night nurse, Gloria, had been at the nurse's station at 0415 when Iris approached and asked her to come look in her room. Iris' door had been partially closed but Gloria saw that it was bright in there. When she opened the door all the way, the bed was on fire. The flames were starting to lick the ceiling.

Gloria started yelling at Iris who was sitting on the floor in the hallway sucking her thumb, "What the hell did you do, Iris?"

"That poor nurse. She told me she ran to the kitchen to get a pitcher of water and realized when she returned to Iris' room that the fire was too big for that amount of water. Gloria was in a bit of shock herself but managed to call the supervisor and the fire department came in no time."

"Did anyone die, Linda? I mean from the fire," Ebony asked.

"No, but there had been a death a few hours before Iris' performance. The nurses had been waiting for the patient's family to drive in from Bakersfield before they prepared the body for the morgue. But when they did arrive, no one could find the body. The patients had been moved to another unit because the smoke had gotten so bad before the fire was extinguished.

"And some of our other patients who were strong enough to walk were mad as hell at Iris. Our one patient, Ralph, found Iris and cursed her out. Gloria said Ralph shook her, 'You fuck'n bitch. What are you trying to do, kill us? We're already dead from AIDS.'

"I don't think Iris really understood what she had done, but I always wondered. She seemed happier that day, like she had just walked down her last runway," Linda said.

"Well, I'll be. It sounds, Linda, like she might have lit the bed on fire for attention. It sure doesn't sound like she was trying to hurt anyone, not even herself, since she left the room and found a nurse," Cal said.

"I agree. And all of us forgot about the fire, especially when she died a few days later. I helped wrap her body. She wasn't mine that day but I wanted to say goodbye to her. Her face looked content.

"Her nurse that day told me she must not have died too long after lunch. She saw Iris enjoying a chocolate milkshake, her favorite."

"That is so sad," Margarita said. "She died all alone."

"True, Margarita. But she must have felt comfortable enough to do it. So many do not, will not, like my patient Stephen from back then," Cal said.

"Would you like to tell us about Stephen?" Linda asked.

"Maybe later, honey. I better get on back to Randy. Some of his lesions could do with some cleansing and antibiotic ointment."

"May I come along, Cal? After I check on Ms. Williams and Ronnie?" Margarita asked. "They're both pretty stable. You know Ms. Williams is off the Dopamine drip and Ronnie's fluids are stabilizing. That vaccine is a miracle!"

"Sure thing, Margarita. You'll be caring for Mr. Humboldt soon enough. This is my last shift, girls."

"Don't remind me, Cal," Margarita said.

JUNE 17, 2021, 6:30 P.M.
National Health Center, Respiratory Unit

Margarita was almost done administering Ronnie Lynch's diuretic when the Secret Service man knocked on the door. "Vice President approaching. ETA 10 minutes."

"Can't wait for the shit show," Ronnie said when the man

walked out of the room.

Margarita laughed a little but said to her patient, "It has been awhile since you've seen your father, Ronnie."

"About a month. They must be back from Greece."

"I'll see you later."

"No, wait please, Margarita. I want him to see an actual Mexican who is legal, professional, and standing next to me."

"You've been doing some thinking, Ronnie, pensando mucho."

"That means a lot, right, Margarita?"

"Bueno, Señor."

Gerald Brugge entered the room. "Good Evening, Ronnie. Margarita."

"Man, I'm really getting the royal treatment now. Must mean I'm getting better or dying," Ronnie said.

Gerald explained Ronnie's father wanted an in-person update on his condition. The White House had called the doctor an hour ago.

"I asked Ashley to be available after I was summoned here. We could not have done any of this without her," Gerald said.

"She's admitting my new patient for me, Dr. Brugge. She's really good with the computer part of it all," Margarita said.

"I know she is. Well, at least she's on the unit," Gerald responded.

Two more Secret Service men came into the room to inspect it.

"Dad has arrived," Ronnie said.

"Hello, son. I take it you are feeling better," the Vice President said when he entered without touching Ronnie.

"I am, father. Thanks to Dr. Brugge and the nurses here."

"*She* is one of your nurses?" Vice President Lynch asked while sneering at Margarita.

"Margarita Ramirez is one of our best and most devoted

registered nurses, Mr. Vice President. We are lucky to have her," Dr. Brugge smiled.

"Hmmm. So, Dr. Brugge, you found the cause of my son's illness. You must have in order to have developed the vaccine. My wife told me Ronnie told her all about it when we were out of the country," Lynch said.

"We did, sir. A pig virus has jumped to humans. We would not have found it, though, without the team of nurses our nursing supervisor, Ashley Smith, brought together. And thanks to your funding we've been able to keep them here over the past several weeks," Gerald said.

"And where did you find such *special* nurses?" The Vice President asked with some sarcasm.

"At the Quilt exhibit earlier this month," Brugge said.

"AIDS nurses? Are there even any of them left?" Lynch asked.

"Enough," Brugge said.

"What did they do here?" Lynch asked.

"They helped us procure the information leading to the viral source in pigs," Dr. Brugge said.

"Ronnie always did like pork. It comes from eating it, right?" the Vice President asked.

While Gerald explained the several routes of viral transmission, including oral ingestion of the infected animal, Ronnie told Margarita, "For the record, I never liked pork and I don't eat it now."

"He doesn't need to know that, Ronnie," Margarita whispered to him.

"So, when is my boy going home, Dr. Brugge?"

"Probably next week. The vaccine has helped him. So far, we have only seen minor side effects. But Ronnie cannot take dialysis forever."

Ronnie said, "I don't want to take dialysis forever. I thought

I could get off of it if the vaccine worked and you said it has, Dr. Brugge."

"Ronnie, I wanted to wait and see if the vaccine helped your disease at all before I discussed the next step with you," Gerald said.

"Am I going to die, Dr. Brugge?"

"I don't think so, not for a long time, we hope, but you are going to need a kidney transplant. Then the dialysis will be able to stop," Dr. Brugge explained.

"No problem there. We'll find you the best kidney to be had, Ronnie, and we'll make sure it comes from the *right* kind of person," Vice President Lynch said.

"I don't give a shit, dad, where it comes from as long as it helps me," Ronnie shouted.

"Mind your lip now, boy. You'll come on home with your mother and me for a nice long rest when the good doctor here says it's OK for you to be released.

"Thank you, Dr. Brugge. You did one hell of a job with all this," the Vice President concluded and rushed out of the room.

Brugge followed him with the hope he could grab Ashley to meet him before he left the unit.

Ronnie was crying. Margarita held his hand.

"What about school? And won't I need a whole bunch of drugs to take for the rest of my life now with a new kidney, Margarita?

"That one night in that bar in Atlanta with that man wasn't worth all this. And I've been wondering if I even really believe in all those things that R. E. Lee believes in and my dad."

Margarita just sat there with him, listening.

JUNE 17, 2021, 7:30 P.M.
National Health Center, Respiratory Unit, Staff Lounge

Ashley Smith was ready to give report on Margarita's new patient, Ted Carter. She had completed the patient's admission after Gerald introduced her to the Vice President of the United States as the manager who staffed shift after shift with nurses who uncovered the origin of the disease his own son had suffered from so much.

As soon as the Vice President left the unit, Ashley asked Gerald if they had enough money for the upscale dinner they had planned for the AIDS nurses tomorrow evening at the Spanish tapas restaurant in the District where Gerald was able to get reservations for a party of eleven.

"I asked for more than enough funds to cover the nurses' salaries, Fred and Thomas' road trip, our vaccine production, the celebration, and any other expenses the nurses might have getting back home. You remember, several of them canceled flights a few weeks ago," Gerald said.

"Smart, Brugge," Ashley said.

"I learned a bit about financial requests back in the day when we still had the National Infectious Diseases Center."

"I bet you did. But how in the world were you able to get all of us in for dinner at Pequeño Paraíso? I've had absolutely no luck getting a table there even for two people and for like two years now," Ashley said.

"Family friend."

"You seem to have them in all the right places, Brugge. I look forward to it. Now I better finish up with this incredibly interesting and very ill patient I have in there," Ashley said pointing to Ted Carter's room.

Gerald asked Ashley if she was wearing a mask with this patient even though the presumed diagnosis was *PCP* pneumonia. Gerald had read something in the patient's chart that made him think it could be tuberculosis.

"Be careful, Ashley. Limit your time in there."

"Yes, doctor," she said with a little smirk and placed her mask on.

Right before Ashley joined the other nurses in the lounge, Ebony had given report on Maria Vasquez with little input from Linda. As Jack Doherty listened to Ebony talk, he kept thinking about someone he took care of years ago at Village Community Center.

"She sounds a bit like an older version of a patient, if me memory serves correct, from 1992 or '93," Jack said.

"Bridgette said she was in your hospital in the early 1990s, but the patient did not remember Bridgette because of the drugs she was on and the toxoplasmosis in her brain," Ebony explained, feeling proud she might have known something Jack did not.

"Bloody hell. That's her for sure, then. Bridgette mentioned her last night but I was too distracted with me own lot to really listen. Like you said, Ebony, Maria Vasquez. I remember now. She was a model. Bone structure looked like old Michelangelo carved her himself."

"That's what Bridgette said, too, well, not the Michelangelo part," Ebony replied.

"It would be hard to forget that one, especially her first time with us. She was in bad shape. A real speed baller to be sure," Jack said.

"It sounds like it was really popular back then," Margarita said. "Cal and Linda taught us all about it today. One of Linda's patients in San Francisco did it too."

"We had quite a few of them down in the Village with us who did. But that was a night to remember when Vasquez came in for the first time. She was bleeding, really hemorrhaging, and we couldn't figure out where it was coming from. She was lying in a pool of it, to be sure."

Jack told them he had asked Ms. Vasquez if she had been

menstruating. The patient was incoherent most of the time from the cocaine and heroin she shot up before she ended up in the ER at Village Community and then on Jack's unit, but she told him and the nursing assistant, Derek, who kept changing her soiled sheets, that she had not menstruated in months.

"We had no reason not to believe her, you know. That kind of drug use usually takes all that away," Jack said.

"Was she shooting up down there, sweetie?" Cal asked and addressed the new nurses in the room. "I know that might seem like a strange one to ask but for those of us who have seen a lot of drug use, that was not an uncommon practice. We sure saw it at Upper East Side Medical, didn't we ladies?" Cal said to Sophia and Sura, who were coming on duty.

"Kimberly," Sura said.

"Yes, Kimberly," Sophia said. "Let me tell you, before Kimberly's dementia got real bad, I found her in the bathroom one night trying to inject a used insulin syringe, she had dug it up from the sharps container on the wall in her room, into her perineum. Another patient gave her the heroin."

"Es eso un cuento, Sophia?" Margarita asked and Alejandra O'Brien, Sura's orientee for the shift, smiled a little.

"No, no, Senorita. I am not telling a tall tale. That one's the truth," Sophia said.

Jack picked up his story again. "She was not bleeding from that. It was coming from the wee baby trying to make its way out. For fuck's sake, we couldn't believe it."

"Oh shit," Alejandra let out and covered her mouth.

"Those were bad times, Alejandra," Sura whispered to her.

"The babe was dead. Small like a pup. Thanks be to God, really. Can you just imagine if the poor thing had lived, having to go through withdrawal, and then eventually death from the HIV she surely had from her mum.

"It was one of the only times a nun came to our unit when

someone died. The babe, you see, needed Baptism to wipe away the original sin, and to set the little one on the path away from Purgatory and to Heaven. Now that's a tall tale for you, a Catholic one, to be sure," Jack concluded.

Sophia, Margarita, and Alejandra laughed.

"Poor, Ms. Vasquez," Margarita added.

"No worries then, Margarita. There's no way she remembers that night. She was in a bad way mentally and physically. I'm bloody amazed, I tell you, she made it out of that time, alive, to the ARVs in the mid-'90s." He paused for a few seconds. "And now she's made it back to none again. Bloody hell.

"Forgive me long windedness, Ebony. Is there anything else I should know about our Maria Vasquez?"

"I think I covered most of the important things, if Linda agrees."

"You did an excellent job, all day long, Nurse Chen," Linda said.

Cal added, "She sure did. So did Margarita. She's a natural with AIDS and KS. Helped me with Mr. Randy Humboldt right after lunch.

"So I suppose I should tell y'all all about Randy. Sura, you and your lovely young nurse here have him tonight, don't you?"

Sura nodded.

"I told Linda earlier, girls," Cal said looking at Sura and Sophia, "that this young gentleman reminded me of someone we cared for back then. First time I've really thought about him in decades. Stephen."

"De Grasio," Sophia added. "Worst KS I've ever seen."

"Me too, even worse than Dr. Greenberg's back on oncology before our unit even opened," Sura said.

"I don't know about y'all, but the longer we are together, the more I keep thinking we are like one grand old Charon

Club. It's a right exclusive one no one would be too eager to join.

"All of us older AIDS nurses, and no disrespect intended for the youngins among us, have had so many memories, so many stories we've been reliving with each other since taking care of these patients with this new virus. And, Lordy be, here's our old one once again," Cal explained.

"Cal, you mean Charon, then, like the ferryman in Greek mythology rowing the dead across the River Styx to Hades," Jack asked.

"'Deed I do, sweetie," Cal replied.

"From what I've heard over the past few weeks," Margarita spoke now, "it sure sounds like all of you have seen a whole lot of muerte."

"And not only saw it, Margarita, but helped them. We had no choice," Sophia said.

"They were on one straight path, without any detours, to the grave. And there were not many nurses who wanted to care for them," Sura said.

"We carried them, didn't we?" Linda began. "We walked with them for their final steps. And, as Cal describes it now, we rowed them to the other side. Made sure they got there with dignity too and as much comfort we could give them."

Cal returned to her report on Randy and then told everyone about Stephen, his beauty, his KS mural, and his family not being there.

"Thank you for that, Cal," Linda said and rubbed her arm.

"But Cal, you said Stephen would not die alone, unlike Iris, Linda's patient in San Francisco. Remember earlier today? How did he die?" Ebony asked.

"I can answer that one, Ebony," Sophia chimed in.

"'Deed you can, Sophia. I just remembered now. You were his nurse that night," Cal said.

"I was just so thankful I was off when Sophia told me all about it. It was not pretty," Sura said.

"Maybe I should wait to tell this one. We still haven't gotten all of the report yet," Sophia said.

"Por favor, Sophia. I'd like to hear," Margarita said and Ebony seconded her motion.

Sophia began where Cal left off. "Stephen De Grasio was really handsome, buried underneath all that cancer. And he was a beautiful being, period. He was so kind to our other patients. As long as he still got out of bed, he helped feed the others who could not eat on their own. He also talked to the patients who never had any visitors. He did not like to be alone."

Cal said, "See, Ebony and Margarita, that's why he wouldn't die alone. Even though he was happy with the way he lived his life. He embraced his KS but . . . ."

Sura took over. "He could not understand why his family could not understand his own satisfaction with it all. Not even his mother did and she adored him, until she visited him. She said he was disgusting, said he would not look like a monster if he had been a good boy."

"That's a terrible thing to hear, especially when you are so ill," Alejandra spoke up now.

"Si, Si, Alejandra. That's one of the main reasons we wanted to take care of AIDS patients back then, so they did not have to hear such ugly things from everyone in their lives," Sophia said.

Sophia continued. Stephen became unconscious late in the evening that last night. And then the bleeding started. His platelets were low as they often were in AIDS patients.

"We called it ITP then," Sophia said to the young nurses.

"We still call it that now," Cal chimed in. "The 'idiopathic' part of the 'thrombocytopenic purpura' acronym some call 'immune' but we still don't know the exact culprit chewing up those platelets."

Sophia told them the KS had to be in Stephen's lungs because he was having a hard time breathing. And she knew that for sure when he started coughing up blood. She told them the night aide, Tom, kept cleaning out Stephen's mouth but he could not stay in his room for too long because they had to care for all of the other patients.

Sura said, "That was another one of those nights when the supervisor left one nurse with one aide on our unit."

"We had our share of them, too, downtown," Jack added.

"How many patients for one nurse, Sophia?" Ashley could not help asking now.

"Anywhere from four to six, sometimes seven. They always felt like those numbers were safe," Sophia said.

"For AIDS patients? That's just simply outrageous! I'm only seeing them now for the first time and I can tell you three AIDS patients is one too many for one nurse. The care is so complex," Ashley said.

"Girlfrieeeend! Did we need you back then," Cal said and snapped her fingers up high. Ashley smiled.

Sophia told them she and Tom rotated running back and forth into Stephen's room in between other patients.

"There was so much blood. The Kaposi's must have eroded a pulmonary artery. It was ruby red. Tom had turned Stephen on his side the last time he was in there. I stepped in a pool of it on the floor. It covered my shoes completely. I yelled to Tom to bring me some surgical booties but it was too late for that.

"He was still breathing. I gave him some morphine and left the room to put on new shoes. I always kept an extra pair of everything in my locker."

Tom had found a mop, she told them, and covered the floor with padding before Sophia got back in there.

"I couldn't believe it. Still breathing, and hard. I gave him another dose of morphine. I sat down next to him. I held his hand. I told Stephen he was safe. I sang to him. God my singing is horrible, but I thought he would like to hear something.

"Stephen liked old Sinatra. The only song I could think of was my mother's favorite.

"Fly me to the moon, let me play among the stars....

"And then he stopped...." Sophia had tears in her eyes. So did Cal and Margarita.

Ashley, Ebony, and Alejandra looked like they had just watched a brutal beating in a movie.

Linda and Sura were staring at the floor.

"This is no way for me to start this kind of shift, raw and exposed," Sophia became stoic now.

"I bloody well know how I'm ending mine," Jack added.

June 17, 2021, 8:30 P.M.
National Health Center, Respiratory Unit

Sophia was thinking about Ashley's report on Ted Carter that had just ended a few minutes ago. She knew nights like this one, starting this way with report pouring over into the first part of the shift.

Sophia's other patient, Ronnie Lynch, could wait for her first visit tonight. He was stable, he did not have dialysis today, and she knew him.

Outside of Ted Carter's room, Sophia ran through what she needed to do: check his oxygen saturation level and check his oxygen tubes and flow rate; collect a third sputum sample for AFB, the tuberculosis bacterium; and give him an Albuterol treatment if respiratory did not make it up to help with the extreme wheezing in his lungs Ashley told her about. The ER doctor might have diagnosed *PCP* pneumonia, but Sophia felt TB after everything she heard.

The patient had lost 20 pounds over the past few months on top of more pounds lost before that. And he lived in the tourist-laden North West district of Washington, D.C., exposed to crowds trekking to national museums and the President's residence.

But what Sophia was most struck by in Ashley's report was the patient's occupation. Ted Carter had been an addictions counselor for thirty years, a milestone Sophia would reach in about six.

The patient's addiction, prior to choosing this career path or it choosing him, was socially unacceptable in a way Sophia's would never be. She thought, no one ever suggests going out after work for a little smack shooting.

Sophia knew all too well, though, that not everyone can stop after one or two drinks, that drinking alcohol with the intent or effect of numbness and amnesia every time is no better than shooting heroin. It's just that Sophia's instrument for substance abuse was a glass, not the needle that, if shared, had placed Mr. Carter in harm's way decades ago.

Sophia washed her hands in the anteroom. She reached for a gown and pulled it over her arms and tied it in the back. Then the mask, an N95, claustrophobic but necessary she knew. They did not have them back then. Goggles and then the gloves. She would wear it all until she assessed how much protection she would need. That was always the delicate balance with AIDS patients: not too much for them but not too little for yourself.

"Good evening, Mr. Carter. I'm Sophia, your night nurse. How are you feeling?" she said her introduction as the door shut with the swift swoosh of a negative pressure room.

"Hello, Sophia. I've had better days. Call me Ted, please," he said panting.

She turned on the light above his head to get a good look at him. He was a handsome Black man, at least he was before the fat cushioning the bones in his face had melted away thanks to the virus' unquenchable thirst to survive.

"Do you have any pain, Ted?"

He shook his head no.

"May I listen to your lungs?"

He nodded his head yes.

After Sophia heard the raucous sound of fluid in there instead of the free flow of air, she explained she would like him to cough up a little more sputum so she could send a third TB specimen.

"How were the first two?" Ted asked.

"Negative."

Ted tried to cough. Nothing.

Sophia placed a few milliliters of saline in the nebulizer chamber and turned it on placing the mask over his face. "This might help us get what we need, Ted."

Dr. Brugge knocked on the door. He still needed to admit the patient.

"Good evening Mr. Carter. I'm Dr. Brugge. How are you feeling?"

The patient nodded his head yes and waved hello as the nebulizer did its work. He started to cough.

Then again. And there it was: the high-pitched ring Gerald had not heard in decades. Now he remembered the ER nurse's note that described the patient's cough as a "whistling sound."

Sophia looked at Gerald and said, "It's been a long time. You have on an N95, right?" She could not see what kind of mask Gerald had on because the doctor stood outside of the lighted area of the room.

"I do. Thank you for asking, Sophia."

Sophia removed the face mask from the patient and positioned the cup. "Please cough one more time and spit in here, Ted." After he did she thanked him and said she would be back.

She placed the lid on the container and exited the room. Gerald followed Sophia into the brighter light of the anteroom.

The sputum was light pink with specks of red in it.

"TB," Gerald said. "TB," Sophia said.

"I'm going to start him on the TB regimen while we wait for these results. The chances of it not being TB are slim," Gerald said.

"Sure seems that way, Gerald. Hey, are you on all night?"

"I am."

"Good. This man seems really sick. Well, you know that. His time is short, I think," Sophia said.

"Whatever you need, Sophia. Thank you for this shift. All of you."

Sophia left to send off the sputum to the lab and to check in on Ronnie Lynch while Gerald examined Mr. Carter and explained the probable diagnosis and treatment he would start soon.

"There are four meds for you to take, Mr. Carter."

"I know two of them. I took them in the beginning. Back then I actually cared about not being able to drink alcohol when I was on them. My priorities, shall we say Dr. Brugge, have shifted seismically," the patient said.

"I will also order more oxygen for you through a mask to help you breathe a bit easier, Mr. Carter."

Gerald finished the physical exam. "I'm here all night."

"Thank you, Dr. Brugge."

June 17, 2021, 9:30 P.M.
National Health Center, Respiratory Unit

Sophia only wore a mask when she opened Ted Carter's door. The patient was walking back to bed from the bathroom.

There was Ed. Ed Arlen, their patient from 1993 and 1994, and then his last admission in 1995 before Sophia left.

There he was, standing up from his bedside commode where he had spent most of his time. Wobbling as he stood, and then shuffling back to bed like an 85-year old ravaged by time. Ed was forty-seven.

There was Ed during that last night Sophia worked. She saw him in the only light coming from the overhead above his bed and the distant bridge providing its moonlight-like glow through the window. Only now did she realize Ed's body was not just prematurely old but that of a prisoner detained for months in a death camp, flesh dripping off of bones.

"Hi, Sophia," she heard him and saw that smile with his teeth devouring his lips. "Sit down and have a peep with me," Ed Arlen had said that night handing her a box of marshmallow chicks sprinkled with yellow-colored sugar, only available around Easter time.

"Hi, Sophia," Ted Carter said now. "I've been spending more time in there than I would like. Are you OK?"

She was back. 2021. "Oh, yes. Sorry, Ted. I was just thinking."

"You've had others like me, haven't you? Lots of them. That young supervisor who was in here before said there would be an AIDS nurse taking care of me tonight."

"Yes, I have, Ted. Now let's get you settled. I see respiratory was here. Your face mask is ready to go."

"They left around fifteen minutes ago. I walked to the bathroom after the Albuterol was done. That's the only time I can really get a good breath, right after that treatment."

"That's good," Sophia said standing next to him straightening his gown and tying the strings on it hanging down his back in loose bows so it would not choke him when he moved around in bed.

"I have your medications. All four of them. You've had these before, right? I mean in the beginning."

"Yes. I had TB in 1989, just like most of the other junkies I messed around with then," Ted said.

"When did you get clean?" Sophia asked him.

"Not long after the TB. That's when I found out I had AIDS. I used heroin since the late '70s. At first, I thought I was just having fun. But then I really needed it. Then I chose it over everything else, my job as a psych tech at the VA Hospital here in D.C., my wife. I lost everything to that damn powder. It's the reason I'm here now."

"You mean because of the HIV you contracted through sharing needles back then, Ted?" Sophia asked.

"Hell, yeah. If I hadn't done any of that, I wouldn't be sick now."

"I guess the other way of looking at it is you wouldn't be sick now if President Rumpel had not stopped insurance companies from continuing to provide coverage for the antiretrovirals that have kept everyone with HIV and AIDS alive, well, and free of opportunistic infections like the TB you have again now."

"Good point, Sophia. You would make one fine counselor."

"Or politician," she said and laughed. So did Ted. "I've been a counselor since 1997."

"I thought you were an AIDS nurse," Ted said.

"I was for a long time but there wasn't much of a need for us, in hospitals anyway, since 1995. You know, hardly anyone got sick after the meds came along. So I went on for my MSW and became an addictions counselor like you."

"What was your pleasure, Sophia?"

"Alcohol. Mainly wine."

"Yeah, I thought I could stay off the heroin if I switched to drinking alcohol but when I learned I had to take that damn INH for my TB, I knew drinking was out. So, the hell with it, I thought. I gave it all up and went back for my Master's degree.

"Actually, I returned to the VA as a counselor. I'd like to think I helped the soldiers who got so fucked up in the Middle East all those years."

"It sounds to me, Ted, like you've had a very rewarding life."

"I have. I even got married again. Sally died last year. We were married about twenty years. I almost relapsed when she left me."

"I did when my husband died. It's hard to know what to do with that kind of pain. People like us reach for the old crutches."

"We sure do. I've realized lately, Sophia, it is not nearly as hard facing your own death."

"I imagine you started thinking about it when you could no longer take your ARVs," Sophia said.

"Yeah. It only took about a month after my last dose for my appetite to go to shit. Lost my taste for everything I loved, especially Italian pastries."

"Like what, Ted?"

"Tiramisu, cannoli, you name it."

"I have a place for you back home in New York," Sophia said.

"Anyway, I started losing pounds as fast as potatoes can roll out of a bag. I was drinking milkshakes, even put ice cream in them. Nothing helped. Just like the old days. And here I am again. I don't know if I'm making it out of this one, Sophia."

"It's so hard now. Without controlling the HIV, the TB, or even if it is pneumonia, is difficult to make go away and stay away. You know the drill. Unfortunately."

"Sure do. I had *PCP* twice before the meds came in '95."

"Ted, have you thought about what you would want to do if your heart stops beating or you stop breathing?" Sophia asked.

"I don't want to do anything. Just let me pass, please.," Ted said.

"Do you want to take the medicine for TB or pneumonia or anything else you might get before that happens?"

"Yeah. Well, unless I start to feel so terrible from the medicine or the disease or any of it. And I sure don't want to take any of those medicines if I'm in pain most of the time."

"You should probably express these wishes in an advanced directive, if you do not have one already, and sign a DNR, Do Not Resuscitate, form so that no one performs CPR or places you on a ventilator," Sophia explained.

"Where's the pen? I need both of them," Ted said.

"I'll get Dr. Brugge to come in for your signature on the DNR and I'll be back soon with an advanced directive."

"Thanks so much, Sophia. I feel like I've known you a long time."

"Me, too," Sophia said and left his room.

JUNE 18, 2021, 12:10 A.M.
National Health Center, Respiratory Unit

It was time for Randy Humboldt's Decadron. Sura thought, as she watched Alejandra program the small bag to infuse over twenty minutes, not all that much has changed. The pumps are different but same principle.

As Alejandra tried to talk with Randy, she could not work the pump, and Sura remembered how hard it was for a new nurse to hang medication or start an IV or adjust oxygen while talking to a patient.

Sura looked at Randy and could see why Cal thought about Stephen, yet she could not get Thomas Mason out of her mind. He was not young like Randy but there was something there that made her think about him.

Sura listened to Randy's lungs and asked Alejandra to do the same. "What do you hear, nurse?"

"They sound clear at the bases but diminished," Alejandra said.

"Good assessment. I heard the same."

Then Sura started talking to Randy about his job. "One of the great things about our nation's capital is the opportunity to work in really meaningful jobs like yours at the CLO, Randy. I remember an older gentleman we cared for. He was a curator at *The Smithsonian*. He only worked on exhibits involving enslaved peoples in the Americas."

"That sounds cool. Very interesting, Sura. How did he end up in New York? Cal told me you two worked together there."

"We sure did. The museum defunded our patient's position once they found out he lived with his younger male partner, a sculptor."

"What year was that, Sura?" Randy asked.

"I think it was 1988. It was early on our AIDS Unit, before Cal joined us. Thomas and Tim moved to New York when Thomas was offered a teaching position, History, at Manhattan University. They wanted to get married."

"And here we are again. After all that time, we finally made it, and now we cannot," Randy said.

"Are you married, Randy?" Alejandra asked even though she knew he had been from Cal's report.

Sura returned to thinking about Thomas Mason. His room was like an eighteenth-century salon with books strewn across two bedside tables he requested and lining the two windowsills.

They always managed to return to the subject of Nazi-ruled Europe. Thomas knew where all the camps were. He said it was one of his special interests. His mother's parents died in Auschwitz. Sura told him about hers in Dachau.

Randy answered Alejandra, "Yes, but she died."

"I'm so sorry," Alejandra said.

Randy was lying there staring, looking lost. Alejandra did not know what to say to move him past this moment.

"You are too young to have lost a spouse, Randy. You deserved much more time. The universe can be so cruel, can't it," Sura jumped in.

"You said it, Sura. Lulu and I were only married a few years. We were just getting started."

"How did the two of you meet?" Sura asked.

"At the CLO. Lulu was the best lawyer we had. She won every case for our transgender clients except her last one when she tried to prove conversion centers were places of hate crimes."

"Well, they are. What happened to her after that last case?" Sura asked.

"They took her away to one. She committed suicide. I never got to say goodbye to her."

"I never got to say goodbye to my brother," Alejandra said.

"Did he go to a conversion center too?" Randy asked her.

"Well, yes, but the other ones for gay people," Alejandra said.

"I haven't met anyone who's been sent to one of them. Well, not yet anyway," Randy said.

"It was bad. I loved Mickey. He was like twenty years older than me. My father's first wife's son, one of eight," Alejandra explained.

"Wow. Are they Catholic?" Randy asked.

"Yes. Irish Catholic. My dad then married my mom like ten years after Mickey's mom died. Never thought he'd have another family but mi mama es Mexicana. Muy Catolico. Very Catholic. So another three."

Sura and Randy laughed.

"How did Mickey end up in one of those places?" Randy asked.

"You know President Rumpel, or Presidente Diablo, as my mother calls him, ordered that database of names to be created from marriage license records."

Alejandra continued to tell Randy that Mickey and his husband Tony had been together at least ten years and were so happy they could finally get married. They were about to adopt a little girl who was found in her home after her mother burned it down. All of her siblings died except one brother who was permanently disfigured by the fire. This little girl, Alice, hid in the refrigerator, she had told the fire department when they found her, because she wanted to stay cool. It saved her life.

"Mickey and Tony fell in love with her. She was like four. They couldn't wait to bring her home. Adorable and a real little pistol," Alejandra said.

"A real survivor," Sura said.

"They never did get her because two officers from the Department of American Values arrested Mickey and then Tony for being gay, for being happy."

Alejandra told them her brother was sent to a conversion center in Philadelphia and Tony was sent to the new local one in Boston. "Mickey killed himself not long after he went in. I'm still not sure what happened to Tony. He's probably dead, too."

"Why do you say that Alejandra?" Randy asked.

"Because they were both HIV positive. Mickey committed suicide when he got *PCP* pneumonia, not long after his insurance stopped covering his ARVs. Tony did not want to live with AIDS either. No chance of that now anyway," Alejandra said.

Randy turned pale.

"Oh no, Dios Míos. I am so sorry, Randy! I did not mean it like that."

"That's the straight up truth, Alejandra. We're all going to die from AIDS. It's like we're on a bad time travel trip back to 1985," Randy said.

"Why don't we let Randy get a little rest now, Alejandra," Sura said. "Do you need anything, Randy, before we go do some other work?"

"No, thank you, Sura," he said.

Sura led the way out of the room and turned off the lights. In the hallway, she told Alejandra she did a really good job connecting with Randy, but her frank honesty at the end of the conversation left the patient feeling a little too vulnerable.

"I feel horrible, for sure, Sura. I need to learn when to stop, to hold back a little," she said.

"You will, sweetie," Sura said and put her arm around the young nurse.

June 18, 2021, 12:20 A.M.
National Health Center, Respiratory Unit

Jack saw Sophia coming out of Ted Carter's room with Gerald Brugge.

"Everything OK in there?" Jack asked her.

"OK is about it. He just signed a DNR."

"He sounded bad off in report, Sophia. Better than hurting him with futile attempts, as you know, love."

"Agree completely. He's damn dyspneic. The Albuterol works for about ten minutes and his breathing goes right back to being labored. You can hear the fluid moving up into his throat now," Sophia said.

"Sounds like the train's coming," Jack said.

"Maybe he'll miss this one. Hey, how's your crew tonight, Jack?"

Jack told Sophia he could not believe how much Betty Ann Williams had improved after the vaccine.

"That's great, Jack. How are the lesions on her abdomen?"

"Still there, to be sure, but receding."

"Amazing," Sophia said. "How's that husband of hers?"

Jack told Sophia Ms. Williams had told him Burt's antibody test for this porcine circovirus was positive. "No surprises there," Jack said. "Then she also told me he hadn't been back round to visit her."

"She must be lonely," Sophia said.

"Not really, truth be told. Her son, Joel, as you know, is a lawyer. Works for the CLO here in D.C. He's been visiting his mum these past few nights."

"That's very nice, Jack."

"Ms. Betty told me it feels good to talk with her son without her hubby being round. The husband's and son's politics are like night and day."

"Yeah, I bet. And I got the feeling when I cared for Ms. Williams that she would be more open minded if she could just be around other people who are. I know Cal thought that, too, in spite of some fairly offensive things Ms. Williams had said to her."

"Now don't even get me going 'bout that Wilson now,

Sophia. I don't know if there's anything in this world that could shake up his ugly, myopic view. Bloody hell, he kept going on 'bout how good it was I'm a 'legal foreigner.'

"For fuck's sake, I have dual citizenship. I'm as American as he is."

"I know it, Jack. Remember Ronnie Lynch was so shocked I was a citizen the first night I took care of him? This bunch of patients will be damn hard to forget, I can tell you that much."

"To be sure."

"Hey, did Ms. Vasquez remember you?"

"She did. Said I looked a little more doughy but remembered me name before I said a word to her. I recognized her straight away.

"Breaks my heart, though, how the past has pulled her right back to uncontrolled infections, the likes of which I never thought I'd see again."

"So true. It's uncanny really. All of us here together seeing all this . . .again. Well, I'm on my way to see Ronnie Lynch. I need a reprieve from my own past right now," Sophia said pointing to Ted Carter's room.

"Break round 0330, Sophia?"

"Only if you find Charlie to make that rock'n coffee of his."

"I watched him the last night I worked with him. Me thinks I can accommodate, love."

June 18, 2021, 1:30 A.M.
National Health Center, Respiratory Unit

Ronnie was talkative. Sophia had given him his blood pressure meds and a diuretic almost an hour ago and she was still in his room. She felt bad for him as he tried to come to terms with the kidney transplant, especially all of the anti-rejection meds he would need to take the rest of his life.

"It's all in the way you look at it, Ronnie. I mean sure it's going to be a drag, sometimes, always having to take so many pills, and you might pick up an infection from time to time. You understand the drugs suppress your immune system so your body doesn't reject the new kidney, right?"

Ronnie nodded his head yes.

"But it sure beats being chained to a dialysis machine three times a week for hours at a time," Sophia finished.

"That's why I like talking to you, Sophia. You give me a different way of looking at things. What you said to me last week about not experiencing life for myself yet has really got me thinking.

"I'm not so sure I feel the way my parents do about a lot of things, especially people. And I'm not so sure I want to go into politics."

"Well, I am proud of you, Mr. Ronnie Lynch, for at least starting to question what was handed down to you," Sophia said. "This is the first step in deciding what's best for you."

"Margarita has helped me a lot, too."

"She's a good nurse and a buena persona."

"That's good person, right?"

"Muy bien, Señor."

"May I tell you something really personal, Sophia?"

"Of course."

"I'm not so sure right now if I prefer women or men, you know, to be with."

"That's OK. No rush. Just remember to be safe when you do have sex. In time, you'll know more about what you want, as you live, as you experience," Sophia said.

"I know one thing, I'll never make the mistake I made in Atlanta. That's what got me here. I mean the sex part."

"I can see that's a tough one to digest, Ronnie. But I also see that being here gave you an opportunity you might not have gotten for a long time in your life, if ever at all," she said.

"I'm gonna miss you, Sophia."

Sophia hugged him and left to go check in on Ted Carter.

JUNE 18, 2020, 3:35 A.M.
National Health Center, Respiratory Unit, Staff Lounge

Sophia knew this needed to be a quick break. Ted was still breathing when she shined her flashlight on his chest, sucking in and out so fast it was hard to count his respirations just a few minutes ago.

"Alejandra, cóma va?" Sophia asked the new nurse as she sat down with a cup of black coffee.

"No tan buena, Sophia. Graciás."

"It sounds like you said it is not going so well, Alejandra," Sura said because she understood enough Spanish to interrupt her. "That could not be further from the truth."

"So, what happened, chicas?" Sophia asked.

Alejandra told Sophia about what she said to Randy Humboldt.

"Well, that is the truth, as hard as it is to believe again," Sophia said. "I guess for Mr. Humboldt's sake, though, you probably should've kept that to yourself. But, damn, Alejandra, I remember saying lots of things I shouldn't have in my first few months as a new grad in the ER.

"I remember an older gentleman who came in with an acute MI and I asked the young lady with him to step out of his sick bay while we started a Nitro drip on him. I thought I was being really supportive as I told her I understood how hard it must be watching your father go through this.

"'I'm his wife, nurse!' Dios Mios she was mad."

"We've all said our share of less than appropriate comments, especially early on in our careers," Sura added. "But, Alejandra, you did a great job of connecting with Randy."

Sura then turned to Sophia. "She told him about her own experiences with her brother and Randy felt so much better."

"Don't you be kicking yourself round, Alejandra O'Brien. You'll find plenty of other folks lined up to do that in this life," Jack said.

"Sophia, I did not mention this to Alejandra but do you know who Randy Humboldt really made me think about?" Sura asked.

"Tell me. You know, I'd like to meet Randy at some point but it's looking unlikely with the way this night is unfolding," Sophia said.

"Thomas Mason, but really his partner, Tim."

"Thomas was that professor we had, right? History, I think. I loved going into his room. I always felt like I was in a little library refuge," Sophia said.

Sura told Alejandra and Jack about Thomas Mason's work as a curator in D.C. "That's what got me thinking about him. Randy Humboldt's work at the CLO here."

"That's right, Sura. They forced Mr. Mason into leaving the museum when they found out he was gay," Sophia responded.

"That's the kind of horrible shite we lived with every day back then, Alejandra. Or shall I say that they lived with," Jack said.

"Sounds like it's back again," Alejandra replied.

"Loco, so crazy, isn't it," Sophia said.

Sura could not remember the opportunistic infection

Thomas Mason had. "I don't think it was KS. But something about Randy made me think about Thomas and Tim."

"I think he had CMV, Sura. He did go blind, remember," Sophia said.

"Oh, yes, yes. Now I do," Sura said.

"What's CMV?" Alejandra asked. "I can't remember that one from nursing school."

"Cytomegalovirus. It seemed to enjoy infecting the eyes, in particular, often visited the kidneys, bowels, and brain, as well. That was AIDS before the drugs came round," Jack explained.

Sura started to think it might be Randy's emotional and financial state that led her down the path of remembering Thomas, but really his partner, Tim. Tim had been HIV positive before Thomas died but he never developed AIDS. He was one of the fortunate long-term survivors, virus carriers whose AIDS switch was never turned on.

"Tim struggled after Thomas died, I kept in touch with him," Sura explained. "He was an antiques dealer but he did not make enough money to live after Thomas' death. He lost the brownstone and he had no access to Thomas' estate. But mostly he was just lost without Thomas in his world."

"Who got the brownstone, Sura?" Alejandra asked.

"I don't know if you remember," Sura turned to Sophia now, "but Thomas had been married in his twenties and thirties. He got divorced in the '70s along with so many of us who began to feel safe and justified in coming out."

"So his ex-wife got everything?" Alejandra asked.

"No, but his two daughters sure did. They fought Tim for that, even though Thomas left Tim everything. Those daughters hadn't talked to their father in years," Sura said.

"And didn't Tim die homeless, Sura? That's what I'm remembering now," Sophia said.

"Practically. He moved into a room in Times Square. But he did not die from any physical disease," Sura said.

"It sounds like he died from a broken heart just like Randy Humboldt will, and most likely before AIDS kills him. He misses his wife and his life with her more than he wants to live now without her. That might be what made you think about those men from back then," Alejandra offered. And Sura agreed.

"Sounds like you've got a good head on your shoulders, Alejandra O'Brien. You're going to make one fine nurse, to be sure," Jack offered.

"It's not just the physical illnesses that have been bringing them back to us now, is it?" Sophia said. "I mean I can't keep Ed Arlen out of Ted Carter's room when I'm in there."

Sophia told Jack and Alejandra about Ed and how different he was from Ted Carter. Ed was not Black, not heterosexual, about twenty years younger than Ted, a jewelry designer not a counselor, and Ed had cryptococcal colitis.

"And then meningitis, right after you left us, Sophia," Sura added.

"Thank you for that, Sura," Sophia said with some sarcasm.

"It was when I saw how thin Mr. Carter is that I started thinking about Ed, but then the way we talked, like we knew each other a long time. That's how it was with Ed Arlen."

"You were so close to him, sweetie," Sura added and Sophia nodded her head.

"Now, ladies, lend me your ears. Forgive me but I'd like to contribute a wee bit to our Club of Charon. What the likes of you have said about your men from the past and the here and now takes me back to 1984," Jack said.

"He was one of the first ones, he was. Ed Rolling."

Jack told them he was also one of the oldest at Village

Community Center. The other patients who were strong enough to walk to the lounge, where Ed sat for hours smoking, called him "Grandpa."

"He came to us from the ICU, a real wee stick he was. A month in there with AIDS and TB will do it to you, to be sure," Jack said.

"That man never wanted to live like that, a bag of bones with a hole in his throat. I mean a tracheostomy, Alejandra."

"I took care of one of those in nursing school, Jack," she said.

"Truth be told, old Ed used to curse the nurse who saved him when he went into respiratory arrest. 'Who the fuck wants to live like this,' he would shout pointing at his throat. At least he could still smoke, and sometimes he took it through his trach."

Alejandra was a little surprised but then smiled.

Jack told them Ed Rolling might seem bitter, or a little angry, from what he said so far, but that was far from the truth. He had found happiness after spending the first few decades of his life married to a woman he loved but was not in love with, and raising a daughter and son who ended up both supporting Ed after he found Hank.

Ed had a successful career as a Broadway costume designer working on some of the biggest musicals, and that's where he met Hank, a dancer.

"Ed told me one night, chain smoking like he did and truth be told I did a bit of it meself back then, too. He said, 'Damn that nurse. I could've been dead. I have my children but my Hank is gone. Died terribly on a stretcher right here in this hospital, in the ER. They didn't have the decency to put him in a room. Hell, no one would even touch his stretcher. God damn that nurse. Why didn't she just walk away? Look at me now.'

"And then he told me something I carry with me 'til this

day. 'You listen to me, Jack, when you're moving through the dark tunnel, you're gonna hear voices trying to distract you and hands trying to grab you. But don't listen! Don't stop! Keep moving toward that light because if you don't, you'll end up right back here again in this hell hole.'"

"My heavens, Jack, I can't say anyone else has ever told me that before. Everyone I have ever cared for that close to death never came back," Sura said.

"Ditto," Sophia said.

"All's I know, ladies, is I'll be keeping me eyes on the light when my train pulls into the station," Jack said.

JUNE 18, 2021, 4:03 A.M.
National Health Center, Respiratory Unit

Sophia was the first nurse to return to the floor. Ted Carter's eyes were half open and he did not stir when she opened the door. She knew he was still alive because she heard the death rattle, the sound of gargling water deep in the throat that doesn't go away with coughing or suctioning or medication.

"Ted, how are you?" Sophia asked standing next to him counting his respirations. 54. Fuck, she thought.

"Ted, how are you?" she shook his shoulder.

"Oh, hello, Sophia. Finally caught a few winks. My chest doesn't feel right."

"Does it hurt?"

"It feels like an elephant is sitting on me. Can you give me something?" he asked.

"I will get some morphine for you after I talk with Dr. Brugge. You have some fluid building up right here," she said as she touched her throat. "Some atropine might help a little with that."

June 18, 2021, 4:10 A.M.
National Health Center, Respiratory Unit

When Sophia returned, Ted did not wake up at all and he was moaning through the gurgling sound.

"You just rest, Ted," Sophia said after giving him the medications through his IV line.

He felt hot. Sophia soaked a washcloth in cold water and placed it across his forehead. She removed his blanket and exchanged the top sheet for a fresh one while positioning his arms on top of it.

June 18, 2021, 4:30 A.M.
National Health Center, Respiratory Unit

Ted did not respond to Sophia's voice or her touch. He was still moaning but the gurgling was slightly less.

Dr. Brugge had entered the morphine orders in the computer for every ten minutes until comfort was achieved as per Sophia's request.

She gave Ted another 2 milligrams through his IV. She checked his pad and saw a small amount of liquid stool there. He was so light she turned him on her own to place a fresh pad there after washing him with some soap and warm water.

JUNE 18, 2021, 4:45 A.M.
National Health Center, Respiratory Unit

Still breathing. The gurgling had transitioned into the sound of inhaling water while trying to force it out but drowning anyway in a murky lake.

And the patient was still moaning but now like a bear shot in the chest, trying to find any position rolling around on the forest floor, that would offer the slightest bit of relief.

She gave him another 2 milligrams of morphine and sat down next to him. She was so hot in her mask, she made a cool compress for her own head after applying a fresh one to Ted's.

JUNE 18, 2021, 4:58 A.M.
National Health Center, Respiratory Unit

Still sitting next to him. He was still drowning. His moaning had softened a few minutes ago but it was back full force, a grunting from the depths of his abdominal cavity.

JUNE 18, 2021, 5:05 A.M.
National Health Center, Respiratory Unit

She was still sitting next to him, rubbing his arm, telling him all about the great bakeries, especially her mother's favorite, back home in the Bronx.

"Those cannolis, I tell you, Ted. You can't find filling like that anywhere. Not too sweet, but just enough, the perfect top off to a perfect lasagna, my mother's of course. She'd kill me if I said anyone else's."

Sophia could see the corners of his mouth move upward,

just a tad. And then the noise stopped.

"You have found peace, Mr. Ted Carter. Thank you for allowing me to share the last moments of your life with you."

She looked at her watch. She texted Gerald Brugge. He said he would be there soon. He was in the pulmonary ICU finishing an admission.

Sophia sat there touching his arm. So fuck'n cold, she thought. Already. After only two minutes. Easy to forget.

Sophia sat there on her mound of shoes that just grew a little higher.

JUNE 18, 2021, 5:15 A.M.
National Health Center, Respiratory Unit

Dr. Brugge walked in with Sura and Alejandra behind him. Sura had seen the doctor walking towards this room and she knew what had happened.

"Sophia, why didn't you ring the call bell?" Sura asked. "We would have been here with you."

"There was no time."

"Time, Sophia?" Brugge asked.

"0507."

"Thank you. Rough last shift. It looks like Mr. Carter was content, though."

"All those cannolis I told him about back home, doc."

Gerald smiled.

JUNE 18, 2021, 5:30 A.M.
National Health Center, Respiratory Unit

Sophia tried to reach Ted Carter's listed next of kin, a friend in D.C. She left a message to call the NHC.

Sura and Alejandra had been performing most of the post-mortem care. Sura showed the young nurse how to roll the shroud under the body, to check for fluids leaking out of both ends every time they turned him, to tie the jaw shut tightly enough so it doesn't drop open and stick in that position when rigor mortis sets in.

Sophia gathered up Ted's few belongings while Sura and Alejandra completed this final act of nursing care.

Jack entered the room with his mask on, looked at the patient, and removed it.

"I was starting to wonder if I was the sole survivor of the bloody apocalypse. I didn't think I was in with Ms. Vasquez that long but when I came out of her room no one was to be found.

"Finally spotted the good doctor and he told me all about Mr. Carter's demise."

Sura and Alejandra were about to cover the patient's face and Jack started to sing.

"Oh, Teddy boy, the pipes are calling . . ."

"I know that song, Jack. My father always sings it when someone dies. It should be Danny boy, right?" Alejandra asked.

"Right as rain you are, Nurse O'Brien." And Jack continued, "The summer's gone, the roses falling . . ."

By the time Jack sang the last line, ". . . sleep in peace until . . .," all the nurses had tears in their eyes standing around Ted Carter's bed, except Alejandra, who was weeping.

"You, Jack, have one hell of a voice," Sophia said.

"They'd kick me out of me race if I couldn't at least keep up with the worst of them," he said.

Jack left and Sura and Alejandra returned to covering the

patient's face and head, but Sophia stopped them and said she would finish the task before calling the morgue.

"You sure, sweetie?" Sura asked.

"Yes. Thank you both. See you in a bit," Sophia said as they left the room.

June 18, 2021, 6:00 A.M.
National Health Center, Respiratory Unit

Sophia thought about the last night she took care of Ed Arlen in April of 1995 and what had led up to that moment. She knew she had crossed the line with Ed somewhere in 1994 when she felt like he had become her friend.

She had asked Ricky if he would like to meet Ed and his partner, Johnny, for dinner at a popular French restaurant on the Upper East Side, not far from Sophia's apartment. Ricky and Sophia were engaged by then but Ricky had kept his own apartment in Battery Park. They both felt a little traditional when it came to living together before marriage.

Ed was happy to finally meet Sophia's fiancé, the Southern lawyer he had heard so much about, and Ricky felt the same way about meeting Sophia's patient, the jewelry designer.

The two couples had a lot in common: a love of Italian Renaissance art, good theatre and food, political views, and the great fortune to have found the best match for each of them.

Deep into the langoustine over steamed green beans, Ed told Sophia he would like to pass on his rent controlled brownstone on 88th and York Avenue to her when he dies, only if Johnny was gone, too, of course.

"He's always trying to kill me off. Like maybe I should start to worry, you know," Johnny said lighting another cigarette and laughing.

"Ed, you're not going anywhere, anytime soon. You aren't either, Johnny," Sophia said.

"Well, I hope not. But let's be realistic, Sophia. My time between visits to the unit is shorter than it was last year," Ed said.

"I could not let you do that," Sophia said.

"Why not? I don't have children. Thank goodness. There's no one else in my family who deserves it. It's only $300 a month. The shittiest room in the Bowery is more expensive than that.

"I want you to know how much I've appreciated you taking care of me, and Sura, of course. You nurses make my stays bearable, even enjoyable, like visiting family you actually like."

Ricky laughed and said, "'Deed, that's always a challenge," Then he winked at Sophia.

"What about the legality of it all?" Sophia asked.

"Well, your hubby to be here is one fine lawyer," Ed said.

"Some conservative-minded judges might dispute that claim, Ed. But, as you know, I spend most of my time defending civil liberties cases, not real estate."

"But, surely, Ricky, you could take a look at the language, or at least show it to another lawyer if you're not certain. My great Aunt Emily's lease remains active with the rent controlled as long as it passes to a family member.

"The exact clause in there, as far as I can tell, does not specify blood relative, just 'family member;' which is why I have spelled out in my will that the lease goes to my business partner, Johnny, the most devoted cousin anyone could ask for."

"Well, there I am, folks, still alive and well, on paper at least," Johnny said.

Sophia and Ricky laughed.

"And I would like the next statement in there to be, 'in the event of my cousin's, Jonathan Bolt, death, the lease shall pass to the next most caring and surviving member of my family, Sophia Maria Lorenzo, the best niece anyone could ask for."

"That sounds good, Ed. I'll take a careful look at it," Ricky said.

"Drag your feet on that one," Sophia whispered in Ricky' ear.

Crossing that line with Ed Arlen did not help Sophia at all during her last shift taking care of him. She was also pained by how much she had upset Sura with her resignation announced two months before.

Sophia and Sura had vowed to stay together until the end, the end of one of them, or the end of AIDS, which they knew was unlikely, or the end of the AIDS Unit. Both of them knew that one was coming when the ARV combinations were close to FDA approval.

And Sophia realized Ed Arlen was not going to make it onto any of them. She could no longer overlook that, as she had been doing, when she saw how Ed looked standing up from the commode.

Sophia also knew Ed was ready to give up living with Johnny gone after his sixth bout of *PCP* pneumonia just a few months ago, not long after a New Year's Eve Sophia and Ricky celebrated with them at the Waldorf.

She ate the peep Ed handed to her after he reached the bed. It was Good Friday night, she remembered. Not that she celebrated but her family had expected her and Ricky at dinner on Easter Sunday.

Their wedding by the Justice of the Peace in Central Park, "an abomination" her mother had called that, was set for the end of May right after Sophia would receive her Bachelor's degree in psychology.

Sophia felt exhausted as she finished eating the marshmallow candy. It was not the exhaustion of a few bad shifts, but came from years of caring for young, sick people who were ostracized by friends, family, and medical staff, who died anyway, no matter how much she gave to them.

She remembered all that now, and how guilty she felt leaving Ed Arlen. Guilty for not caring for him ever again, for not being there when he left for good. And guilty about how much she would miss his advice to her about how to make up with Ricky when they had a fight or how to tell her mother things she did not want to hear.

There had been no guilt with the other patients that last night, no sadness she carried deep down inside like she did for Ed.

"Sophia, you will have a great life." She remembered his last words. "As a counselor, married to Ricky. He's a good one, you know. And as a resident with your new husband of my brownstone for the rest of your life, if you want. You've been there. It's cozy but spacious. And location, location, location, girl."

Sophia had laughed and wrapped her arms around Ed. She knew he had felt twice that size at New Year's. "I'm going to miss you," she told him.

Sophia was looking at Ted Carter's face trying to remember what had happened next after that last shift on the AIDS Unit, after saying good bye to Ed Arlen.

She closed the shroud and walked out of the room.

June 18, 2021, 7:45 A.M.
O'Toole's, Crystal City

Sura invited Sophia to breakfast with her and Linda at their hotel but Sophia chose the more robust atmosphere of this pub with Jack and Alejandra.

"Here's to me River Liffey back home in Dublin. I like to call it the River Lethe, though, because I forget about me troubles walking along it. May the same happen to last night's shift," Jack toasted and he and Alejandra gulped down their shots of whiskey.

"Sophia, you've had the worst of shifts, to be sure. A wee dram of goodness is well-deserved, love," Jack said not knowing Sophia's history.

"You are so right, Jack," Sophia said and ordered an Irish coffee. She then raised the mug when Jack and Alejandra drank another shot.

Sophia savored the sweet, pungent smell of the whiskey deep down inside the ceramic vessel. Not too far from Lethe myself, she thought. Dios mios. This is exactly how it began after my last shift back then.

Sophia had stopped in to say goodbye to Ed Arlen after she gave her final report, something she never did before or since. Report was supposed to be the final curtain call for the shift.

She remembered it so well now. It started with a coffee, just like this one, but at O'Grady's on Madison Avenue, a popular hospital bar where nurses and doctors and respiratory therapists and pharmacists ended their shifts.

That coffee led to another, and another and then to a bottle of wine carrying Sophia right on through to lunch where she only took a bite of the pub's signature burger.

Sophia had been awake for twenty-four hours at 4:00 P.M. that Saturday, Easter weekend 1995, and it was her first drink since before she met Ricky.

"Ricky, Holy fuck!" she shouted out from the sink of her bathroom trying to wash away the stink of her last shift mingled with the alcohol.

She was supposed to have dinner with him, a quiet one

before the big Lorenzo Sunday Easter celebration.

"Rick, it's Sophia," she was leaving a message on his answering machine. "I'm not feeling so pwell. I need to cancel. Love you." She knew that did not come out clearly.

She made it to her bed and passed out for a long time. God dammit, that was bad, she thought sitting at O'Toole's bar wrapping both of her hands around the mug and inhaling the smell of the whiskey. Jack and Alejandra were laughing with some ER nurses they met, and both of them were now drinking herbal tea.

Sophia never made it out of bed until the late morning sunlight pierced her eyes that Easter morning.

"Fuck'n shit!" she yelled. She saw several messages on her answering machine, two from Ricky and one from her mother.

Sophia wanted more to drink, so Ed Arlen stayed away, and so she did not have to deal with Ricky or her family after getting drunk.

She did not keep any alcohol in her apartment but she knew where the closest liquor store was on 3rd Avenue, two doors down from the pizzeria.

Before she opened the bottle of Chianti, Classico Reserva, she said, "Fuck it! If I'm going in, I'm going in good." Then she called Ricky.

"Are you alright, Sophia? You sounded awful last night," he said.

"Yes, Ricky. I'm sorry. I can't do my family today. It's been rough, since my last shift."

"I thought it would have been good for you, good for us, celebrating the last one together last night. Too late for that now, but it's OK. Maybe we could just have a quiet dinner together today."

"I can't, Ricky. Not right now."

"It sounds like you need to call your sponsor, Sophia.

Kathy, right?" Ricky said.

"I'm fine, Ricky. I'm sorry," she said and hung up the phone.

She called her mother next.

"What do you mean you can't do Easter, Sophia? Are you OK?" Mrs. Lorenzo said.

"Just feeling a bit under the weather, Ma."

"What about Ricky?"

"He'll be fine. I'll call you soon,' Sophia said and hung up.

Sophia was embracing the mug at O'Toole's.

When she woke up that Easter Monday she had a horrible headache and a feeling of drenching nausea. Then she thought, "I don't have to do this. I have the power to be grounded, to stay sober. It's been two and a half years now. I have Ricky, my family, a few good friends, a bachelor's degree completed, and grad school on the way."

She called Kathy later in the day in case she had worked last night in the ER.

"I fucked up, Kath," Sophia said when she picked up the phone.

"When did you start, Soph?"

"After I got off duty Saturday morning, my last shift on the AIDS Unit."

"When did you stop?" Kathy asked.

"Last night. I put in a movie and finished the second bottle of wine. I felt like I did not want anymore."

"That's good, real good, hon. Now find a meeting tonight. If you feel like a drink tomorrow morning, go to another one. At the very least, hit a meeting once a day every day this week. Call me tomorrow.

"And listen, Sophia, don't worry about anyone else until you feel strong enough inside to make any contact."

"Thank you, Kathy. Love ya," Sophia said.

Sophia pushed away the mug now and texted Dan Napolina. "Hi, Dan. When's the next meeting at that Catholic church?"

One minute later she heard a ping on her phone. "Hey, Sophia. 0900. Do you want some company?"

"Yes," she texted back.

JUNE 18, 2021, 10:15 A.M.
The Little Crystal Deli, Crystal City

Sophia and Dan were eating bagels with cream cheese, sesame for her and everything for him, while Dan sipped coffee and Sophia drank tomato juice so she could get some sleep today before the dinner tonight.

Late yesterday morning, Sophia had been walking, and walking, around Crystal City in order to get tired enough for a few hours of sleep before her last shift.

A few blocks from the hotel, she noticed a Catholic church that looked at least a century old but she knew it could not be since this city was relatively young. Circling around the outside of the church, she searched for the date and found it engraved above the main entrance: 1965.

"Well, it is pretty old after all. The year I was born," she said out loud and smiled a little.

And then she saw some people coming up the steps from the church's basement, including Dan Napolina. That's when she realized they shared more than similar family backgrounds, careers, and dead spouses.

"Well, what do ya know. Fancy meeting you here, Sophia," Dan said.

"I had no idea, Dan. I actually envied your ability to only drink one glass of wine every night like you said, and did at dinner last Saturday evening. And just one nightcap, as you put it, that first night we were all at the Crystal Nightingale."

"I never did order that one," he said.

"That's right. Now that I think about it, you had water instead."

"Until last night when I got off duty. It all went to shit, real fast. I should've seen it coming. My search for that nightcap before my first shift was all about my memories coming back, anticipating the new infectious disease we were gonna be facing.

"But then it went fine, normal for me anyway until last evening. Having to take care of that poor kid with KS. I know you haven't been back yet, but we got two of 'em last evening," Dan had told Sophia walking together yesterday.

"Yeah, Sura told me last night after Ashley called her and asked her to come in and orient one of the new nurses."

"It brought back so much, Sophia. I tell you. My one Chianti I prided myself on having every evening since 2011, blew up in my face. I had a whole damn bottle and finished that off with an Amaretto cream coffee.

"First thing today when I woke up, I found a meeting. I hadn't been to one in like a year."

Sophia continued walking with Dan and told him about her own recovery without giving too many details.

Until now, sitting here at this deli after her last shift at NHC. She told him again, like she had told the small group at the meeting, how she let go of that Irish coffee in front of her, clenching it most of the time, smelling it on and off for like twenty minutes, and then pushing it away and texting him.

"I gotta tell ya, Sophia, you got balls. No offense, if you know what I mean."

Sophia laughed.

"I couldn't do it. The first sign of old AIDS, I was drinking like I wasn't an alcoholic, well not like a recovering one anyway."

"I get it, Dan. It all came back to me too. My last shift on our AIDS Unit in New York, my patient then who I was way too close with, and not knowing what to do with eight years of that kind of pain when it was all over. Taking care of Ted Carter last night transported me right back to 1995," Sophia said.

"Another one came in?" Dan asked.

"Yeah. He *was* so sick."

"He fuck'n died on your watch, Sophia?"

"He fuck'n died on my watch, Dan."

"And you didn't take a drop of booze?"

"Not a drop. I came so damn close."

"Like I said, balls. Well, Sophia, you should eat up. You need some rest before tonight."

JUNE 18, 2021, 7:30 P.M.
Pequeño Paraíso, Washington, D.C.

As Fred listened to Sophia's story about Ted Carter, he went from sipping his sangria to gulping it.

"Damn, did I miss a lot, Sophia. I haven't been on duty since earlier this week and now I'm feeling guilty for gallivanting around the South while you've been wrapping dead bodies again."

Sura heard Fred and chimed in, "Technically, I did the wrapping," she said and hugged Sophia.

"Look, Fred. You deserved your time, especially after making that trip down to Georgia with Thom. We couldn't have confirmed the source of the virus without you two."

"Hey, how's your father-in-law, anyway?" Fred asked because he had heard all about Tucker Abbott owning the farm where the infected pigs were sold to their patients.

"Just fine. Thanks for asking. So tell me about your Southern adventures," Sophia said.

"I went to Charleston and Savannah. Beautiful, just beautiful," Fred said. "Other than the heat."

"I've never been. I would have tagged along with you if I had known you were going. I could have returned early for my last shift," Sophia said.

Ashley heard her and said, "And what a horrible one it was for you, Sophia. When I heard what happened to Mr. Carter this morning after you got off duty. I should've never asked you to work last night."

"I'm a big girl, Ashley," Sophia said.

"Balls, big balls, I tell ya," Dan whispered in Sophia's ear.

Sophia smiled and said, "Ashley, what I mean is, that's very kind of you but I am just fine."

"Damnnn, girl," Cal said sitting across the table from Sophia. "You rowed across another one? Only you and Sura have that kind of strength."

"And luck," Sophia said.

"I only helped after the fact, Cal. Sophia did all the hard work," Sura said.

Bridgette only heard what Cal said and asked Sophia, "You had a death last night?"

"I did, Bridgette."

"He was damn lucky to have you," Bridgette said.

"Thanks, Bridgette," Sophia said.

"Charon Club, honey. It doesn't stop," Cal said.

"Now I really feel lost," Bridgette said and Fred agreed.

"It dawned on me this week. There are, there were, not

many of us who helped our patients back then, you know, reach the other side," Cal said.

"We sure did. No one else would, or could, or even wanted to," Bridgette said.

Jack was standing behind Bridgette now with a fresh glass of sangria. "Cali here, you see, summed it up for us, gave it to us in a nice wee package, Bridgette, during shift report last evening, to be sure.

"She said, We're all members of this here Charon Club," Jack finished.

"Oh, I get it. Like the ferryman in the underworld carrying the dead across the river. Greek mythology. Holy shit. That is what we did," Bridgette said.

"And all of us together now, these past two weeks, we've shared our memories, our stories about them," Cal continued.

"And you know, Cal," Sophia said taking a sip of Orxata, a nutty, milky, non-alcoholic drink that pared well with the patatas bravas she was eating. "It just struck me. Now for the first time in our lives, as we've relived these memories of our AIDS patients and shared them with each other again, or for the first time, in my case really, it's like we're still Charon. But we're taking a return trip."

"I hear what you're saying, Sophia," Dan said now. "We're rowing them back to life, their stories to the world of the living, to us anyway, but to other nurses, too, who weren't there, like Margarita, and Ashley, of course."

"And Ebony," Cal said.

"And Alejandra," Sura said.

Fred added, "Can't say back then I would've volunteered to be a member of a club like this."

"That's why I said what I did yesterday, Fred. Well, you weren't there, but I said it's an exclusive club but it sure ain't one you'd want to get into," Cal said.

"Let me finish, Cali girl. I may not have volunteered back then if I had known what the life long side effects were going to be, but I'm damn proud to be a member of this club in hindsight," Fred said.

Thomas joined the nurses now after he finished his conversation with Gerald Brugge about the specific clinical trials he had worked with in Philadelphia.

"What am I missing, Frederick? I still enjoy a tame club now and again," Thomas said.

Dan explained what they had been talking about and then said, "Bet you never thought we'd be in the same club, Tommy boy. I'm just kidd'n ya, Thom."

Thomas smiled. "I told Fred and Linda last week that I've felt like it is finally time to let some of the past breathe."

Linda added, "You put it much more eloquently than that, Thomas. He said cashmere served to keep his memories covered up for years, but he was ready now for a lighter fabric, to let them breathe."

"I hope you chose Mulberry silk, Thomas. The finest there is," Cal said.

"Obviously, my tastes are not as sophisticated as yours, Cal," Thomas said.

Everyone laughed.

Gerald Brugge stood up so everyone could hear him. "There are two types of paella coming out soon, seafood and vegetarian."

"This is unreal. All these tapas dishes are so delicious. I'm stuffed already," Fred said.

Sophia agreed as she took another bite of tortilla, made with potatoes and egg.

Ashley took another bite of fried bread saturated with chorizo and said, "I never heard of Migas before I went to Barcelona, and this Migas tastes just like it did there."

"I couldn't agree more, Ashley," Sophia said. "And thanks for reminding me of the name. I loved the food there, too."

Sophia and Ashley talked for a while about their trips to Spain.

"It must be so nice living in Florence, Sophia. You are a train ride instead of a plane ride away from such great art and food, just pick your country," Ashley said.

"It is wonderful. The only drawback is not seeing my family as much as I would like," Sophia said.

When the large plates of paella were set next to the table on large round wooden racks, Gerald stood up tapping a spoon on his sangria glass.

"Thank you, just thank you, nurses. You were the best type of nurse back then, and each one of you has been absolutely invaluable these past two weeks. It was an honor and a privilege. Ashley, please, the stage is yours."

"All of you make me so proud to be a nurse. It's only been a few weeks but it feels like I've know you for years. Margarita will never forget this time, and Ebony and Alejandra will not forget their first shift, your last one.

"Please remember as long as I'm at the NHC, all of you will always have a position. Thank you for what you did," Ashley finished with her eyes welling up and sat down.

"Ash, I can only hope you now know a little bit more about the world before 1980," Dan kidded with her.

"I'll have you know, Nurse Napolina, I've been streaming old Bugs Bunny and Daffy Duck cartoons in the morning, before work," Ashley said

"That's when they actually showed them on TV for us as kids. You like 'em?" Dan asked.

"I do. They're well done, for sure," Ashley said.

The owner of the restaurant, Mia García Lichtenstein, walked over to the table after one of the waiters she assigned to the special guests to assure excellent service told her they were done eating.

"Mia, this was superb. Thank you," Gerald said and kissed her on the cheek.

"My pleasure, Gerald. I am glad everyone enjoyed," the owner said and then gave Sura a big hug and kiss.

Gerald leaned around Ashley and asked Sura how she knew Mia. Sura told him all about returning to *The Holocaust Museum* after she heard Gerald mention the Lichtenstein name the evening when all of the nurses met there, and about discovering that Lenny is her first cousin on her mother's side.

"Mia is Lenny's youngèst son's wife. I met her this past week at one of Bonita's wonderful dinners," Sura said and then asked Gerald how he knew Mia.

"My mother, Sura, and Mr. Lichtenstein were childhood sweethearts, if you could even use that term in that awful place," Gerald said.

"What an incredibly small world we occupy, Dr. Brugge," Sura said.

"It really is unbelievable. My mother got out of Dachau with one of my great aunts and they made it to Flanders where she met my father, eventually. My dad became a doctor and always wanted to practice medicine at a major cancer center in the States. I was born here," Gerald explained.

"Did your mother find my cousin, Lenny, again in D.C.?" Sura asked.

"Yes, at *The Holocaust Museum* when the shoes were here in 2004. My parents were visiting my wife, Myra, and me. They still lived in Boston then. My father died a few years after that.

"I've kept in touch with Mr. Lichtenstein ever since my

mother introduced us, and even more so after she died last year."

Ashley had been listening to their conversation and said, "See, Sura, you now have 'family', not just 'family friends' in all the right places," nudging Gerald's arm and smiling.

The sound of a flute and light drums floated in from the band room next to this private dining area.

"That's right nice," Cal said.

"It sounds like the call of the Sardana," Sophia said.

"Oh, I loved that when I was in Spain, Sophia. Danced to it every chance I got," Ashley said.

"Let's go check it out, Sophia," Cal said.

Gerald told them the Sardana band from Barcelona was on tour across North America.

"Did you arrange that one too, Brugge?" Ashley asked.

"Not on my own," Gerald replied.

"Family friend," Sura and Ashley said at the same time and laughed.

Several plates of Churros and warm dark chocolate dipping sauce bowls were set on the table as the nurses started making their way to the music.

Sophia grabbed one on her way. "Deliciosa," she said.

Dan Napolina ate one and then approached Gerald. He asked the doctor if Mrs. Johnson's antibody test results were back yet.

"Just saw them this morning, Dan. Thanks for checking. Negative," Gerald said.

"Good news for her, at least she has that. So look, doc, it was great working with you. You're a real good one. You really give a shit."

Gerald smiled and Dan went into the next room to listen to the band.

Cal ran back into their dining area when she remembered

the card she had in her purse for Gerald. It was a thank you with the website address of Sansvir's new product, HIB (herbal immune booster).

They were alone and Cal said, "Gerald, I don't know how much you know about the activist group, RLA."

"Right to Live with AIDS, right?"

Cal nodded.

"I learned my lesson about paying attention to advocacy groups back in the day," Gerald said.

"Well, what's in here is hot off the presses. You can get your own supply for your patients or just pass the information along to them."

Gerald opened the card. "Thanks, Cal. I'm glad you trust me with this. This is the link to the ARVs, right?"

"Deed it is. It has been a distinct pleasure working with you, Dr. Brugge," Cal said and hugged him and then hurried back to the dance floor.

Gerald joined the big circle of nurses dancing to the festive music.

Sophia said, "What a perfect conclusion to our time together. AIDS nurses, and one of the doctors, performing the danse macabre."

"That's intense, Sophia," Ashley said in step with the music. "The paintings I've seen show skeletons dancing."

"We're not there yet. That's something to celebrate," Dan said.

"Hey y'all," Cal raised her voice leaning into the circle. "Let's keep our club going, as long as we can."

"We could meet somewhere in the world, every now and again, couldn't we then," Jack said.

Everyone nodded their heads, and danced and danced and danced.

PART 5

KEEP ON ROWING

June 23, 2021
Train from Washington, D.C. to New York City

The rain was punching the window as the train treaded through the storm in its northern quest. Sophia was glad for the reprieve from the North Carolina sauna-like days she had just spent with Ricky's family.

She had rented a car in Crystal City after a light breakfast with Sura and Liz at the hotel the morning after their big dinner. It felt like 1995 all over again, saying goodbye to Sura, hoping not for too long this time.

How long had it been? Sophia remembered thinking when she turned onto the long, graveled road after an almost six-hour drive. Three years? No longer. That's right, I never did make it down here to see Tucker before I left the country in 2017. Christmas 2016. Too damn long.

And it dawned on her as she drove through the dust from the Abbott family's farm road, that she would not be coming here at all if she had not begun to reckon with the emergence of her own insecurities when the going got rough with men in her life. It had always been easier to just blame them and leave.

Like she had done with Ray, the only guy besides Ricky she kept around for longer than a few months. She had bumped into him at a downtown club about five years after high school. He was an editor at one of the big publishing houses.

Their two-year romance ended, though, after another night filled with too much cocaine, for him, and too much alcohol, for him and Sophia, in a Brooklyn loft whose occupants they did not remember meeting.

Sophia told Ray the cocaine was preventing their relationship from becoming more meaningful. Ray offered that Sophia's drinking might be playing a part. She broke it off after that. No looking back.

But Ricky was different. She knew she did not want to walk away, ever. Sophia had worked up the nerve to call him two days after Easter 1995, when she achieved sobriety again with some confidence.

Ricky was a little pissed when he arrived at the diner. Why wouldn't he be? Sophia thought then. I did ruin the holiday weekend. He kissed her on the cheek instead of the lips after she stood up, but he rested his hands on both of her shoulders and said, "I'm glad you called, Sophia. Now tell me what in the hell happened."

She told him all about it. The last shift, Ed, Sura, and all the drinks.

"You should have called Kathy Saturday morning," he said.

"No shit. I know that. I don't need your judgement. I have enough of my own to last me a lifetime."

"All I meant, Sophia, was a call to your sponsor might have prevented the binge or maybe shortened it."

"I'm sorry I can't be perfect like you, Ricky," she said with sarcasm.

"That's a hot one. I lapsed after Steve died from AIDS in '91. I couldn't take how horrible he looked lying in that bed. I felt terrible it didn't happen to me, too. I drank for a week, took an emergency vacation to do it," Ricky said.

"I didn't know that."

"No, you did not. You also don't know how much I admire you for taking care of AIDS patients all these years. All that wasting away, all that sickness, all that death. To be perfectly honest, Sophia, I don't know how you haven't stayed drunk all of the time."

She laughed. "Thank you, Ricky. I thought you were judging me."

"Not in a million years, darling. We're all broken to some degree. The sooner you accept that you are, too, the easier you can be on yourself and on me when I suggest something for your own dang good."

The rain was lighter now as the train neared the next stop in Philadelphia. Sophia was thinking about first seeing Tucker when she reached the house this past Saturday. He looked a little older but was still tough as nails, pushing a wheelbarrow filled with pig waste.

She felt glad, so happy, to have found Ricky Abbott, the only man who really understood her, accepted her for who she is, someone she lost way too soon. But at least she had him.

She smiled now as the train moved out of the station into the attenuated sun setting in a mud-streaked sky. Her father-in-law made beans and rice with "jalapenos just for you, Sophia," he declared, along with baked chicken for dinner after she arrived.

"Bueno, Tucker, Bueno. Gracìas."

"Denad, as you say, Sophia."

"Close enough," she said with a smile.

After dinner drinking strong cups of coffee, Tucker asked

her what happened during her time at the NHC. Sophia focused on how good it was to help with a new virus and to see some old nurse friends and meet some new ones.

"So, Tucker, I never did ask you if your blood was positive for antibodies to the PCV."

"Deed it was. Not surprising at all with the way I hunker down with my pigs. Bad batch of the vaccines last year. That's what that Dr. Durante from the CDB told me. Said it was on account of how warm it was out in the Midwest where the vaccines are produced.

"I tell you what, Sophia, if we don't start paying attention to the damage we've done to our good Mother Earth, we're gonna have to move into caves to not burn up. Thankfully, I'll be dead before it comes down to that."

Sophia laughed and said, "Maybe not, Tuck, maybe not."

"So, darl'n, you never did tell me how those men got so sick from the litter I sold to them."

"Well, it turns out Tucker, most of them crossed their foreheads with the pigs' blood."

"Lordy be. They sound like they might've been a little sick in the head themselves."

"That's a good way of putting it, Tucker."

The New York City skyline was moving in closer and closer. Sophia felt the calming familiarity of her first home, as she left behind her intermittent one in North Carolina, and anticipated the return to Florence while the turbulence of the emotional landscape she had traversed over the past month percolated deep down inside of her.

Late July, 2021
Mount Vernon, New York

"I can't believe you're going back to Italy already, Soph," Terri said taking another bite of tiramisu and a big sip of espresso at the Lorenzo home.

"I've been here two months, Ter," Sophia said.

"Well, it doesn't seem that long. You had other things going on, like taking care of dying AIDS patients again. What the hell are the chances that would've happened?" Terri said.

"Boy, they really find ya, don't they, the freaks, ya know," Diego said joking.

"Stop fuck'n calling them that, Diego," Sophia said. "It was an honor caring for them again."

"What you had to deal with, Sophia," Mrs. Lorenzo spoke now. "I thought those days were finally behind you."

"It looks like they're never going to be, Ma, at least not the memories," Sophia said.

"I'm so proud of you, for not slipping," Mrs. Lorenzo said.

Terri shook her head in agreement and Diego added, "Yeah, me too, sis. You're a tough one."

"By the way, Ma, the lasagna was excellent," Sophia said.

"I'm glad you liked it. Now tell me something, Sophia, are you going to see that nice man again who came to take you to dinner the other night? I heard you two looked very comfortable together at Anthony's on Arthur Avenue."

"Yeah, Ma, you've always had a direct line to Antonia. If it wasn't for her cannoli and Anthony's manicotti, I would've suggested another restaurant for us to eat in. But I knew Dan would appreciate their food before returning to L.A.

"Hey, wait a minute, Sophia. I didn't hear about dis one. It only took ya like two decades to even go on a date again. It's about time, heh. What does he do?" Diego asked.

"He's a nurse. I met him working at the NHC."

Mrs. Lorenzo added, "And an actor. I couldn't believe my eyes when I opened the door the other night. He looked exactly like an older version of that Tony, the son on that series from way back about the family on Arthur Avenue."

"Get the hell out of here. *The Amicis on Arthur Avenue*. I loved that show. You're dating the brother, sis? Way to go," Diego said.

"It's the last real acting job Dan had, Diego. It got him through nursing school, though," Sophia said.

"That's something, isn't it. Tony from *The Amicis*," Diego said.

Terri's wife, Leslie, added, "I think it's nice, Sophia, really nice that you met somebody like you, another caring person. And like Ricky in that way, too."

"Thanks, Leslie. I don't know where it will go. I'm not really sure where I want it to go."

"So, are you going to see him, Sophia?" Mrs. Lorenzo asked again.

"I told him if he's ever in Florence, to look me up."

"Auntie Sophia, I hope we see you in Firenze," Sophia's niece, June, said after climbing into her lap.

"Who taught you that Italian, June? You sound good. Bene, that's Italian for good. Bueno, that's the Spanish," Sophia said.

"Grandma did," June replied.

"Well you and your mamas are always welcome. Bienvenido, that's Spanish for welcome. Benvenuto, that's Italian. Anytime at all," Sophia said and hugged and kissed her niece.

JANUARY, 2023
Florence, Italy

The snow was starting to stick to the statues in the Piazza della Signoria. Sophia liked to walk home this way from her therapist's office on the other side of the Arno.

Although Sophia was content with her work as a counselor, her friends, and her ability to pop off to Amsterdam or Paris for long weekends, she was beginning to feel like she might want to visit the States, too, especially after Dan Napolina spent some time in Italy this past Thanksgiving. They explored the Amalfi Coast, the birthplace of the Napolina family, and Sicily together.

That's why Sophia continued in her sessions with Anya, at least every two weeks, to deal with her fears about death. Sophia always figured if she never got too close, she never had to deal with that kind of loss again.

But she was beginning to think that passing up an opportunity to love again just might be more painful than a possibility of dealing with death.

Anya had been helping Sophia open the secured shudders she had locked around her heart years ago while also encouraging her to visit the old AIDS days more frequently than she did so the pain was not as great.

Sophia found those visits, though, really could only occur with Sura. She had promised herself she would contact Sura at least once a month. And she did, either through texting or emailing.

And she called Sura on special occasions. Talking inevitably led to one of their ferry rides from the past, like the one they took during their Hanukkah call last month.

"Sophia, sweetie, thank you for calling," Sura said then. "How's the weather in Florence?"

"Mild for now. How about the Big Apple?"

"Raw. But we have a few inches of snow on the ground. Real powdery like the night that one hospital guard found our patient walking outside on Madison Avenue in her gown and boots. Do you remember that, Sophia?"

"How could I forget? We never did figure out where she got those boots."

"But we sure did need them. She wouldn't budge when we tried to walk her back inside," Sura said.

"That's right. We got Tom to help us pull her, to slide her back in on her feet like she was skiing," Sophia said.

They both laughed.

"She was a nice lady. Frida, I believe was her name," Sura said.

"I think that's right. She was Mexican. I remember now. She never stopped looking for her son, Pablo. 'Donde mio hijo?' she would yell out. That's what she was doing out in the snow that night," Sophia said.

"The virus in her brain never gave her the amnesia she so desperately needed," Sura said.

"Pablo died a year before she got ill. Right, Sura"''

"I think that's right, sweetie. Anyway, the snow here tonight. . . ." Sura changed the subject.

Sophia was going to call Sura's wife, Liz, to wish her a happy birthday right after she got home from therapy tonight, but she was delayed in the Piazza by a sound she normally would not have heard if the snow had not muted pedestrian noise.

It was a faint bark. She looked on the ground next to the *David* statue and saw a white dog wrapped in a red blanket. The little dog was shivering looking up at Sophia.

"My heavens! You poor thing!" Sophia let out.

Now the dog barked again and leaped up off the ground to

stand next to Sophia.

Sophia bent down and moved the dog's head looking for a collar and some tags.

"You couldn't possibly be feral. Your blanket is too pretty and your fur is too smooth. How could anyone leave you?" Sophia said out loud as she picked up the dog.

San Valentino, 2023
Florence, Italy

She lit one candle for Ricky sitting at the table with the dog in her lap. And then she lit another one for all of her AIDS patients.

One thing was clear to Sophia: she loved Davinia. That's what she had named the dog after she brought her home that cold night.

Sophia had notified all the dog rescues and placed lost and found signs with the dog's picture all over Florence. No one called. No one claimed her. By the third night with her, Sophia had hoped no one would, and now she could not let the dog go if they did.

The vet said Davinia was around one year old and in good health. Abandoned puppies were not an unusual occurrence in Florence, he had told her.

It was cold tonight. Sophia made some tomato soup and an egg to top off Davinia's dog food. She sat down to watch some news with a blanket that Davinia made her own.

"The President of the United States of America has been arrested for crimes against humanity," the female British broadcaster announced as two guards from the Global Human Rights Council, the GHRC, escorted Rumpel out of the Oval Office on the TV screen.

"What the hell! Oh my God!" Sophia set down the bowl of soup on the coffee table and jumped up from the couch. Davinia started to bark.

She called her sister. She knew it was around 3:00 P.M. in New York. Terri would be at work but she always had her cell phone close.

"Ter. What the fuck is going on?"

"They finally got the bastard," Terri whispered.

"How?"

"Let me call you back in about an hour, Soph, when I'm off."

Sophia sat back down on the couch and listened. A South African ambassador visited Las Vegas this past New Year's Eve. He dined in an Alvin in Wonderland dinner theatre in one of the most popular casinos on the strip.

The show for the holiday featured five Mexican immigrants shot dead with rifles by the paying customers and five more guillotined by big Vegas rollers. The ambassador notified the police immediately. The chief said they were aware of the entertainment and would take care of it.

When no one visited the ambassador for a statement that night or the next morning, he alerted the GHRC Headquarters in Geneva.

The news broadcaster continued. An investigation was launched and it was confirmed that President Alvin Rumpel indeed owned and operated ten Alvin in Wonderlands across the nation where undocumented Mexicans were killed during the shows every night. This was Rumpel's unofficial immigration control policy.

"Unfreak'n believable," Sophia said to Davinia. "We only knew because Fred and Thomas took that trip to Georgia and Margarita told Cal all about the casino her family worked in in

Delaware. But who would have ever thought the rest of the world would know. Fantastico!"

Davinia barked again.

Sophia called Dan Napolina knowing he was off work today.

"Hey, Dan. It's Sophia."

"How are you, Sophia? How cold is it there?"

"Around 40 degrees Fahrenheit but it feels 30."

"How's that new dog of yours?"

"Snug as a bug on my blanket."

"Hey, Sophia, have you heard about that no good bastard?"

"That's why I'm calling, Dan. I guess Vice President Lynch will take over, at least until the election this November."

"It's coming on in a minute, the swearing in, Sophia. Trying to find a good channel. Found it. Look for the curtain in the Supreme Court building. Ya know, the red curtains behind the pillars."

"Hold on a sec," Sophia said while clicking the remote control. "Holy shit! That's Ronnie standing there," Sophia said when she found the channel Dan had on.

"Yeah, I kinda remember his face. I was only in his room like once or twice," Dan said.

"He looks much better now. Really good, actually. And look at that pretty girl with him," Sophia said.

They both listened now as the reporter said the soon-to-be President Lynch's son, Ronald, was in attendance with his fiancé, Alessandra Alvarez, a fellow political science graduate student at Thomas Jefferson University in Alexandria, Va.

"How great is that, Dan! Not only did Ronnie choose not to pursue the same path as his father, for now anyway, but he's in grad school where you're faced to at least question the world. And he's engaged to that Peruvian girl he told me about when I took care of him!"

"That's nice, real nice. Hey, so, Sophia, now that things are starting to look up here, how would you like to visit sooner than later?"

"I sure would, Dan, Ciao. We'll talk soon."

LATE FEBRUARY, 2023
San Francisco, California

Cal sent an email to Sophia, Sura, Jack, Bridgette, Thomas, Linda, Fred, and Dan.

Dear Charon Club,

I promised y'all that we'd stay in touch. I hope none of you thought for a minute that it would only be by email. And if so, you can see how tardy I've been in my intent.

This June is the 40th anniversary of the first AIDS unit opening at Bay City General Hospital, as we know the very first one, Linda and Fred's old unit.

The Quilt will be here for the month, well, at least the California panels, which is more than enough for us!

Let's try to get together for a week, or at least a few days, whatever you can manage, especially now that our country is beginning the long journey towards restoration. How does the week of June 5 or June 19th sound? I am sooo booked the one in between those two.

P.S. I can block some rooms at The Hudson Hotel in Pacific Heights. Swanky, swanky, swanky!

Keep on rowing,
Cal

AFTERWORD

In August of 2018, I finished reading a new novel about AIDS, sitting next to my sister, Wendy, on the beach, sipping a Bloody Mary.

"I think I'm going to write another book on AIDS. I can't believe I'm saying this, but I think I have to."

"Not surprised at all, Gina," Wendy said through a hesitant smile.

It took me six years to write my non-fiction book, *Plague-Making and the AIDS Epidemic: A Story of Discrimination*. I needed to examine, post mortem, the awful treatment experienced by all of my AIDS patients, by everyone who had lived with the virus and then died from the disease in the U.S.A. before the discovery of the antiretroviral drugs in the mid-1990s.

And I thought I had said everything I needed to say in that book until that summer when I read Rebecca Makkai's *The Great Believers,* about a Chicago gay male arts community devastated by AIDS during the early years and the aftermath decades later experienced by all of the survivors.

AIDS fiction usually focuses on East and West Coast artists and urbanites. Makkai's story is not a traditional one, nor is the story about AIDS nurses. But how unusual, I thought as I closed her novel, that no one has ever written a novel about those of us who worked on AIDS units in the 1980s and 1990s.

We were there, close enough to understand our patients' pain, their suffering, their fears as they struggled to live and then die from a virus that we knew did not choose them because of who they were. But the world outside of their hospital rooms, transformed into cocoons of safety by us, as we cared for them week after week, month after month, thought very differently. And we dealt with that ugliness, too.

That novel had not been written, I realized, because it needed to come from one of us. And I knew if I was going to be the one to bring it forth it would mean going back, reliving those memories again, of the AIDS unit I worked on in New York City from 1987 through 1994.

I wanted to get us right, though. I wanted to capture what we do as nurses, what we had to do back then. And I wanted to capture the West Coast nurses' experiences, too. What was different? What did we share as we cared for those within the miasma of discrimination on the opposite ends of our country?

I had to go to San Francisco, where it all began, to the first AIDS unit, 5B, that opened at San Francisco General Hospital in 1983. Of course, I knew it was no longer there: none of them were, thankfully.

I flew west in March 2019 reading *The Joy Luck Club* for the fifth or sixth time, the perfect choice for this journey.

I had been fortunate enough to correspond with Tim Wilson, librarian and archivist at the San Francisco Public Library, when I discovered the 5B archives were housed there. The West Coast AIDS nurses had been smart. They kept records.

And I read through all of them, especially what the 5B nurses called their "Remembrance Book," a large diary, a ledger of the patients they cared for, cared about, who all died from AIDS for too many years.

Tim Wilson put me in touch with Alison Moed, one of the original 5B nurses. It felt like we had worked together back then as we shared our stories over dinner.

I had been thinking about the narrative structure this novel would take before I went to San Francisco. How could I tell our story in a way that would appeal to readers outside of the medical profession? How could I get these nurses back together again to relive the past in the present so the world could see how we survived, carrying those who suffered from AIDS with us?

Creating another viral outbreak seemed to be the way to go in early 2019. I did not know then that a second coronavirus was lurking behind closed doors. I searched for a virus that theoretically could jump to humans from other animals, like HIV did, but had not and probably never would. I wanted the virus to cause similar syndromes, like HIV does, and to initially infect a group of people who most nurses would not want to care for, even AIDS nurses.

But they do care for these patients as they come back together again, sharing their stories from the old days while allowing the reader to witness what it means to be a nurse, to be humane, especially today.

I decided on the chronicle form, not only because my medieval graduate studies background begged me to do it, but also because I hoped it would make it easier for the reader to absorb the nurses' memories about the old virus as the quest to find the new one and its cure unfolds.

This fictional chronicle would also serve, I hoped, to unite the shared experiences of East and West Coast AIDS nurses.

And ultimately it would be an homage to Randy Shilts' *And the Band Played On*, the original personal, political, and medical chronicle of the AIDS epidemic that beckoned and then confirmed my move into AIDS nursing in 1987.

The nine AIDS nurses in *The Charon Club* are fictionalized composites of fellow nurses and people I worked with and knew back then. There is a lot of me in Sophia, for instance, but also other strong nurses I was fortunate enough to know and become friends with are there, as well.

I hope if any of the 3NE and 11E crew finds this book in their own quiet corner of the world they have a right good laugh alongside any tears.

The memories in this novel are primarily my own, dispersed across my characters. Many of them are embellished, just a bit, but too many of them are not at all.

I wrote the novel from July 2019 through October 2020. It was painful emotionally. Then politically it started to feel like a picture of Dorian Gray as COVID-19 tiptoed its way across the globe and our president appealed to the basest of beliefs as he polished the tumor of racism into the shiny stone of patriotism.

I am so fortunate to have had colleagues at that time who listened to me as we tried together to make sense of it all, to figure out why it felt like we were on our own dark train.

That train has derailed, at least for now. But that does not mean we should ever forget or ignore the ramifications of any oppressive political system. The 20th century Holocaust across Europe is a prominent presence in this novel because it felt like we AIDS nurses lived through one. And this history of AIDS should not be forgotten.

The greater part of my gratitude goes to Lisa Kastner and Running Wild Press for recognizing the importance of this story and delivering it to the world. Abigail Efird's editorial enthusiasm, gentle support, and genuine interest eased its passage. Without your publication, general readers would have little insight into the more unpleasant, but necessary, work we nurses do, and nurses in our current COVID pandemic would never be able to witness those of us who also cared for people rarely discharged home with their families. Pandemic nursing has consequences indeed, providing surprising rewards alongside persistent defeats.

I am fortunate and grateful for the time Tim Wilson, and especially Alison Moed, gave me out in San Francisco, and to the attentive library staff at the History Center at SFPL.

My parents, Penny and Denny, and my sisters, Wendy and Michelle, lived through those years with me, listening to my stories about my patients, and I know how horrifying it was for them at times. But they did it anyway. And then they relived all of it with me again, including my brother-in-law, Joe, as I wrote this book. Thank you, just thank you.

My husband, Mike, did not live through those days with me but he has had the distinct displeasure of reliving them with me during the writing of my first AIDS book and now this one. His love, his emotional and intellectual support, especially in always being my first reader, kind and stern at the same time in his editorial and narrative commentary, have enriched my life in ways I never could have imagined, and I cherish him every day.

Our dog, Wat, entered our lives during the last year of my writing *Plague-Making* and years later was by my side and in my lap for most of the writing of *The Charon Club*. He has reminded me that life and literature are so intertwined, so impossible at moments to disentangle.

Wat died after a long struggle with diabetes in early August

2020 as I was writing the final death scene in this novel. That's when my own already too large mound of shoes grew even higher.

ABOUT THE AUTHOR

The Charon Club is Gina Bright's first novel. Her short stories have appeared in Sundial Magazine, The Copperfield Review and Zoomorphic. She wrote a non-fiction book, *Plague-Making and the AIDS Epidemic: A Story of Discrimination* (Palgrave Macmillan, 2012), years after working on an AIDS unit in New York City. Gina has a doctorate in medieval English literature and enjoys her work as a registered nurse caring for oncology patients in Norfolk, Va., while writing every day and traveling again with her husband now that the world is opening back up again.

RIZE publishes great stories and great writing across genres written by People of Color and other underrepresented groups. Our team consists of:

Lisa Diane Kastner, Founder and Executive Editor
Mona Bethke, Acquisitions Editor
Rebecca Dimyan, Editor
Abigail Efird, Editor
Laura Huie, Editor
Cody Sisco, Editor
Chih Wang, Editor
Pulp Art Studios, Cover Design
Standout Books, Interior Design
Polgarus Studios, Interior Design

Learn more about us and our stories at www.runningwildpress.com/rize

Loved this story and want more? Follow us at www.runningwildpress.com/rize, www.facebook/rize, on Twitter @rizerwp and Instagram @rizepress